Arthritis:
THE NEW
TREATMENTS

WITHDRAWN

Arthritis:
THE NEW TREATMENTS

Julian Freeman, M.D.

Contemporary Books, Inc.
Chicago

Library of Congress Cataloging in Publication Data

Freeman, Julian.
    Arthritis, the new treatments.

    Includes index.
    1. Arthritis.   I. Title.   [DNLM: 1. Arthritis—
Popular works. WE344F855a]
RC933.F72   1979   616.7'2   79-50975
ISBN 0-8092-7344-6
ISBN 0-8092-5960-5 (pbk.)

Copyright © 1981, 1979 by Julian Freeman
All rights reserved
Published by Contemporary Books, Inc.
180 North Michigan Avenue, Chicago, Illinois 60601
Manufactured in the United States of America
Library of Congress Catalog Card Number: 79-50975
International Standard Book Number: 0-8092-7344-6 (cloth)
                                    0-8092-5960-5 (paper)

Published simultaneously in Canada by
Beaverbooks, Ltd.
150 Lesmill Road
Don Mills, Ontario M3B 2T5
Canada

Dedication

Somehow, dedicating a book on arthritis didn't seem quite right, so this book isn't dedicated to anyone. But I would like to thank Stephennie and Heather for their help and patience.

Contents

This book has been prepared solely as a source of information and ideas concerning arthritis and its treatment. It is not intended and must not be used as a medical guide for the treatment of any medical problem. Drug names and usual dosages have been included only as a matter of general information. These are not intended as, and must not be used as specific recommendations or prescriptions for use in the treatment of any medical problem. This book and the information in it are not intended as a replacement or alternative to proper and customary medical treatment and advice. The author, publisher, and all others connected with the preparation of this book assume no responsibility for actions or treatments undertaken based on information in this book.

Unlike the physical sciences, medicine has no basic principles or laws of nature that have withstood the tests of hundreds or thousands of years of time and experiment. Any area of medicine, including the treatment of arthritis, is an area of on-going research and rapid change in ideas and treatments. Because of this, *Arthritis: the new treatments* can't be a final statement of the best and only treatments for your illness. Many of the treatments in this book are quite new. Some won't be available until the mid or late 1980s. Particularly with these recent treatments, remember that the full range of their dangers and benefits, and the real effects of their long-term use can't be known at this time. As new information comes to light, the opinions and ideas on the causes and treatments of arthritis may have to be changed.

How to use this book

If you're reading this book to learn about arthritis, begin by reading the entire first chapter, regardless of what you're looking for. From there you can go through the book in several ways: If you know what kind of arthritis you have, you can proceed straight to the chapter discussing your problem, and then to the final chapter on general considerations and treatments. Of course, I wouldn't object if you read some of the other chapters along the way. If you don't know what you have but don't want to spend much time, there is a section in each chapter on what each type of arthritis is like. These are listed in the index under "characteristics." Look through these until you find one that fits. Then read the first section of the *last chapter*. This gives a quick guide for distinguishing the different types of arthritis. Then go back and read the chapter on your type of arthritis, and the sections on the look-alikes for that illness. Of course, if you have the time or interest, go ahead and read the whole book.

The index to this book is very unusual. The book itself has almost no medical or technical terms in it. However, you're bound to run into these terms, and want to know what they mean. Since you won't find them in the actual text, they are in the index, which will refer you to the common name given in the text and index.

Introduction

THIS BOOK IS DIFFERENT FROM ANYTHING YOU'VE EVER SEEN ON ARTHRITIS. It tells you what you can do about arthritis that will really work. It also tells you what is coming in the next ten years, what to look for and the new treatments which are good for you to use. It tells which treatments are just a waste of your money and time. But, more than that, it tells you why you can expect a treatment to work or fail; how to determine for yourself whether some new treatment you've heard about is any good or not. The whole story is in everyday terms so you can understand it. No medical words or technical terms, except those you'll need to discuss what's really going on in your body with your own doctor.

If you're a young person—under 20 or 30—and your joints hurt or your muscles ache, this book is for you, too. Arthritis does happen in young people. If you aren't sure you even have arthritis, this book is still for you—by the time you've read it, you'll probably be able to tell for sure what you have and what you don't have.

If it hurts when you get up in the morning and you can't move because your muscles are stiff and your shoulders ache with each step, you may begin to think you have arthritis and are getting old. You start looking for a cure and relief from the pain. You may even wonder why it hurts when you get up—why should a person under 70 have arthritis? When you look around for answers and relief, you find hundreds of drugs, vitamins, and treatments that are all supposed to help or cure the problem. None of them really seems to work. You try to read about arthritis and what to do for it, but you get buried under an avalanche of books and articles that don't tell you much, except to eat bran or take vitamin C. Others may give some pertinent information, but they use so many medical words that you can't make sense out of it all.

The story behind arthritis isn't simple. If you want to understand it and understand what's wrong with you, you have to know why arthritis happens and why the treatments work. If you understand the general plan of things and how it all works, the details are easy. Suppose I asked you to remember this line of letters and repeat it to me after a few days:

O T T F F S S E N

If you try to memorize it, chances aren't too good that you'd remember it. If I told you to repeat the first letter of each number from one through nine, that list of letters would be as easy as One, Two, Three.

This book works like that memory trick. From beginning to end, it starts by giving you the basic keys for understanding arthritis, why it happens, and how to treat it. Regardless of what your problem is, start with Chapter One on what arthritis is and how it works. *Almost all arthritis is the natural result of the way our bones and joints are made and keep themselves going.* Once you understand how they work, it'll be easy for you to follow why arthritis begins and gets worse. All treatments for arthritis that are worth anything work in definite ways. There's nothing magic about them. They all do something specific to the way bones or joints operate. Once you understand what's going on, you'll understand what treatments will help you, and which ones won't.

Suppose you don't know if you have arthritis, or what kind it is, if you do have it. Start with Chapter One, too. If you want to help yourself, you must determine what's wrong first. There isn't any magic pill that cures all illnesses or even one that relieves all types of pain. Which remedy works depends on the cause of the problem. Since there are lots of pills and treatments around, you're better off first determining what's wrong and doing the right thing the first time, instead of the last. If your joints ache or your muscles feel more stiff than you think they should, chances are you have arthritis.

The following chapters, except for the last one, discuss the different types of arthritis and the treatments to use that really work. If you know what type of arthritis you have, you can proceed directly to the right chapter. If you don't know, your best bet is to read this book through. If you're in a hurry, look in the index for the sections of each chapter that discuss the characteristics of different types of arthritis. Then read the chapters of the one or more that seem to fit what you have. Finally, read the last chapter on treatments in general for arthritis. Even though each type of arthritis has its own treatment, all the treatments have a lot in common, and you will profit from knowing the overall picture on treatments for all types of arthritis. It's like painting: If you paint your bedroom, you need a different type of paint than you need to paint a boat. Still, knowing how to paint in general helps in painting almost anything. Knowing something about how to take care of arthritis in general will help you ease the pain and take care of the specific type of arthritis that you have.

This story of bones and joints may sound useless to you, but remember that most types of arthritis begin in how our bones and joints were made before we were born. Most other types of arthritis come from the way our body does or doesn't take care of infections we get.

Arthritis:
THE NEW TREATMENTS

1

Where it all begins

THE MOST COMMON TYPE OF ARTHRITIS is arthritis of aging, or what doctors call *osteoarthritis* (arthritis of bone). This type of arthritis is caused by the way bone keeps itself in shape. It may seem strange that the way bone fixes its damaged and broken pieces is the cause of arthritis, but unfortunately, that's the way it works. In addition, the same thing that causes the arthritis of aging plays a part in the worsening of other types of arthritis as well.

Bone is like a skyscraper. It has a skeleton like the steel beams that make up the framework of the building. On top of this skeleton a marble-like cement is laid down, both on the outer walls and along the inner halls and offices as well. There are two differences between the bone and the skyscraper: The first is that, in bone, the entire cement work, marble, and steel beams are constantly being remodeled. The second is that, in a skyscraper, the steel beams give strength and support to the building; the

1

outside and inside walls are just room dividers and a protection against the weather. In our bones, it's the opposite. The "steel" framework provides some bracing against bending and stretching, but not much support and strength. It's there mostly to tell the body where to put the cement. The marble is what provides the real strength. Why is our body set up this way? Why not have just one structure that never changes? First of all, we grow and as we grow our bones must change their basic shape as well as their strength and thickness. Otherwise, the stress we put on them would go the wrong way and our bones would break like toothpicks. Secondly, we do occasionally break our bones. More often, although we don't usually realize it, we cause tiny cracks to form here and there in our bones. These hairline cracks as well as the large breaks must be repaired. Our bones must be able to make patches. Making a patch in bone means that one broken end has to literally fuse with the other. The fused parts must end up in perfect alignment and position. If not, the weight and stress will be wrong and the weld will soon give way. As with metals, to fuse the bones and then gradually realign them, the ends must be melted down. The only way this can be done with a marble-like material such as bone is to actually take the cement apart bit by bit, put in new steel beams, and lay new marble on top of them. This is exactly what our bones do. But this is also a bit-by-bit remodeling process.

Let's look at the details of this. The "steel structure" of our bones is more like a cage-like weave of ropes, all joined together. The cords are made up of several strands that wrap around each other. They bend easily, but don't stretch much. The lengths are joined end to end and are occasionally interwoven side to side as well. Each of these strands serves as a "seed" for the laying of a marble-like cement along its length. Gradually, minerals (calcium, phosphate, and fluoride) and water from our blood combine along the lengths of these strands to form a marble-covered rope. In a short time, so much marble is laid down along the rope that each little cage that's formed becomes a solid block of reinforced marble. All of these are tied together by the rope to form hard, long columns in the bones. These columns give the bone its strength and hardness. The rope within them protects somewhat against bending and stretching. When the bone remodels, it starts by removing the marble along the rope. Once the rope is clear of marble, it can bend and change its shape a little. If a lot of change is needed, the rope itself can be removed or squeezed over and a very differently shaped column is laid down. Since the original rope framework is still there, the remodeled column links up to the old ones, and the overall structure is strong and solid.

Here, your body is actually a spongy piece of material, like foam rubber, that can turn itself into a piece of stone. Then, if it must, it can become like foam rubber again, change its shape, splice itself together, and turn back into stone. That's a pretty neat trick, but how does your body tell the ropes where to go? What even weaves them in the first place? It's all done by a central controller. This is a living cell—one of the basic units of the living stuff your body is made of. The controller lives at the center of a tiny cylinder of rope and marble, having surrounded itself with strands and lengths of rope, like a spider in its web. The controller can also produce chemicals that cause the marble to form from the minerals in the blood. At other times, it releases other chemicals to dissolve the marble as easily as paint remover dissolves paint.

How did the controller get there? It was put there as our bones grew, in many instances before we were born. As our bones were growing when we were children, a "wave front" went with the joints as they moved farther out on the end of the bone. The controllers were deposited along the way. They remained, made their cages of rope and

BONE GROWTH

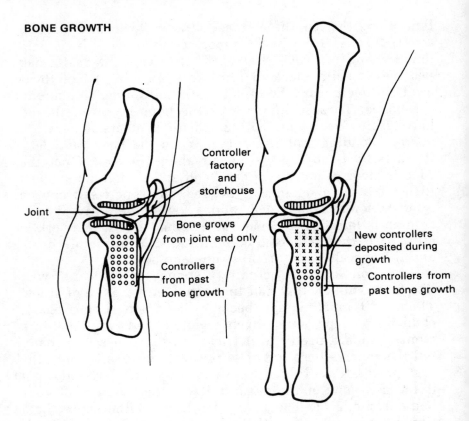

cylinders of bone, and maintained and remodeled them as they went along.

That's how the controllers do their work. What tells them what to do and when? Electricity. The bone sets up an electrical charge of several thousand volts when you stand or press on it. The voltage is greatest along the long section you press on. So when you stand or when your muscles pull against the bones, a very strong electrical force is set up along the line of the pressure. With voltages this high, the controllers have no trouble telling where to lay down more marble and rope. The presence of this electrical force is what tells the controllers where not to remove the existing stuff, as well as where the new material should go. When the bone is broken, the electrical force is lost immediately. At the broken end, in response to the loss of electrical force, the controllers release

ELECTRICAL FORCE ALONG LINE OF PRESSURE DIRECTS CONTROLLERS

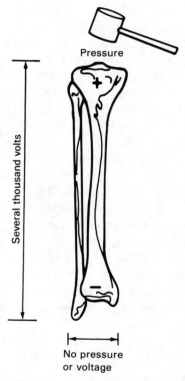

Pressure

Several thousand volts

No pressure
or voltage

chemicals to dissolve the marble, remove the rope, and make way for a weld to form. The central controllers also release chemicals to cause pain and swelling that goes along with the break in the bone. Once the weld is made, the whole bone is reshaped, using the electrical force as a guide. It isn't often that a bone breaks all the way through. Much more often hairline fractures form instead. These are very small, and may only partially crack a cylinder of marble, or may crack into a quarter inch or less of the bone. Even these cracks, that you can't see, are repaired because of the loss of electrical force they cause in the bone. This way the bone keeps from weakening with time.

If you take a piece of most metals, like steel, iron, or aluminum, and bend it back and forth, the metal breaks along the bend. The break occurs because, as you bend the metal, tiny cracks form in it. These cracks get bigger as you bend the metal more. With real marble and similar rocks or glass, it's even worse. All you need to do is scratch the surface and bend the stuff slightly with a sharp blow. This enlarges the cracks so fast that the material just breaks off. In your bones, having the rope inside the marble helps prevent this, but if the tiny cracks that form aren't repaired quickly, the same thing happens in your bones, too. The fact that it doesn't means that each controller is feeling the electricity in the bone properly, and making repairs where it should.

The controllers aren't perfect in their repairs. Mistakes they make show up after a period of decades as arthritis of aging, or wear and tear arthritis. This arthritis is the result of the controllers removing too much bone at the area just under the joints and not putting enough back into the crystal pattern. The joints have Teflon®-like caps on them that seem to rely on the electric force from the bone below to stay in condition. With a poor repair, this force is less than it should be and the teflon cap also falls into disrepair. This weakened electrical force is the main factor in wear and tear arthritis. The basic problem starts before you're born: it's in the way the controllers do their job. As their mistakes add up and the electrical force progressively weakens, arthritis sets in. For most people, it takes 60 years or so to show up. In a few people, it takes much less time; in others, much more. If you've damaged a joint in an accident, the controllers have much more repair work every day just to keep things together. *As they work, their mistakes add up faster, adding the arthritis of wear and aging onto any other type of joint damage, including other types of arthritis. In addition, some of the chemicals released in the joint itself by these other types of arthritis cause the controllers to remove more bone near the joint.*

Unlike wear and tear arthritis, most other forms of arthritis are not a result of a problem in the bone itself. The problem is usually in the joints. So, let's go over how the joints are put together, what they do, and how they keep themselves in good shape. Then, we can better understand what causes other types of arthritis, and what the other treatments for arthritis really do.

First of all, think about what your joints actually do. Remember that most of your body is made up of solid bones that don't bend or twist. If we are going to do anything—talk, walk, bend, use our hands—these bones must move. At the same time they must remain attached to one another and not separate. In order to do that, most of the bones are tied by cables in a way that allows them to swing in one or several directions while they are attached. It's like a lid swinging open while hanging on a box. Lids use hinges for this. Look at a hinge closely. You see that these are made from two metal plates with knuckles that have holes in them. A metal pin runs through the holes to keep the plates together. The lid swings open and shut by having one plate swing on the pin, while the other plate stays in place. Our body can't use a joint made like a hinge. The pin won't take the strain that the joints in the body have to take. There's no way to *continuously* lubricate the pin, or keep it from wearing out. It's difficult to make a hinge that lets the lid move freely in several directions.

To avoid these problems, our body uses a completely different type of "hinge" design. Most of our joints are similar to the "mated surface" and "ball and socket" joints. A few are "flexible joints." In the mated surface joints, the ends of the two pieces have surfaces that are smooth and polished. Where they meet, the pieces are also partially rounded. The rounding can be in the opposite direction on each piece to prevent slipping out of contact if the joint has to hold much weight. It's used in places where one of the bones has to move in many directions. This is the ball and socket joint, or ball joint for short:

The rounding can also be in the same direction. This is

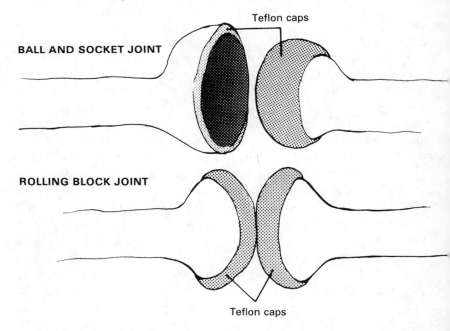

the rolling block joint: This allows for easy movement in *one direction only,* and works well if the weight supported is directly above the joint, but not off to the side. Finally, some joints are called flexible joints. A piece of plastic-like material that can withstand frequent bending over a limited range links two bones together. This type of joint is useful where not much movement from any one joint in a string of bones is needed, but where the joint itself gives structural support to something. On the ends of the bones that form the joint is a smooth slippery material somewhat like Teflon® which causes little friction. In addition, this covering absorbs lubricant from the joint. This further cuts down on friction and wear, and makes this material self-lubricating. The Teflon®-like covering has the medical name, cartilage. To keep things simple, and to remind you of what it does, it will be referred to as teflon throughout the book. This covering is made by cells like the bone controllers that sit just under the joint, at the base of the cap. These cells are continuously producing more covering at the end of the bone to replace what's worn out as the surfaces move' and rub. We don't know at this time if the teflon also has electricity within it, and we don't know for sure what tells its cells to make more of it. Unlike the marble in the bones, the teflon is not a crystal, but seems to be a glass: a liquid that is so thick and slow-moving that it appears solid most of the time. Glass can't have electrical forces in them that are made by pressure alone, the way crystals can. The teflon's controllers probably get the message from the electricity in the bone underneath the teflon cap. Perhaps this tells them how much teflon to make to keep the joint in shape.

There are a few other important parts to the joints. The joints I drew for you, especially the rolling block type, have a real problem: they tend to fall apart. To prevent this, the joints are held together by strong cables similar to the ropes that reinforce the bone. But they're much larger and stronger. These cables go across the joints both at the center, deep inside the joint, and along the outer borders in the rolling block joints. In a few joints, like the knee, there are even special pads of teflon to both absorb the shocks and keep the two parts in proper position.

The joints are surrounded by a watertight bag, deep beneath the skin. This bag starts below the joint and is completely glued with leakproof cement to the bone below the teflon cap. The bag stretches across the entire joint and is glued to the other bone in the same way. Besides keeping unwanted stuff out of the joint, the bag also seals in a special lubricant. The lubricant is like an oil in the joint. It's there to cut down on friction and neutralize things that could harm the joint. Most oils can be squeezed out from a joint if the two parts are under a lot of pressure. The joint lubricant won't do this: It sticks to the surfaces even under extreme pressure. In addition, the teflon cap acts like a sponge, picking up this oil from the joint sac when it isn't under pressure. When the joint is under extreme pressure and has to handle weight, more oil is actually squeezed into the area of contact from within the teflon, rather than squeezed away. Ordinarily only about 5 or 10 drops of oil are in the joint bag. The rest is soaked up in the teflon cap. By putting a constant amount of fresh fluid in the bag at all times, the joint is constantly changing its lubricant. The old lubricant isn't as good as the new, since it breaks down with time and use. The constant changeover keeps the oil in good shape.

The bag surrounding the joint has a fine lining that connects with the arteries and veins in the rest of the body. The lining, using materials it takes from tiny arteries, produces the lubricant. The teflon caps don't produce any lubricant themselves, but pick it up from the bag. If the joint is damaged or infected, the lining produces a somewhat different type of lubricant and in greater quantity to protect the joint and help to heal or fight the infection. If enough fluid is pumped into the joint the sac swells. The lining of the joint performs another important function. Every now and then, a piece of the teflon cap flakes off or the cables that hold the joint together may fray a bit. If these bits and pieces of teflon or cable were left in the joint, the tiny bits of teflon or cable would wear away at the caps like so much sand. To prevent this, the bag's lining has garbage collecting cells that pull in the bits as they come in contact with the lining. They also collect any bacteria and viruses that might infect the joint. At the same time, they take in some of the lubricating fluid and break it down, to make room for the new stuff. If the joint has a lot of undesirable things in it, some are released into the joint fluid to do the collecting and return to the lining when they have completed their job.

All the joints I've talked about so far are joints that move. There are a few joints in the body that don't move, but get arthritis nonetheless. The flexible joints, which are constantly being bent back and forth, don't get arthritis in the usual sense at all, though they do wear with age. Since it isn't a true arthritis, problems with these joints don't get much attention in this book. Most of the joints that don't move are in the pelvis, a very large set of bones which forms the entire area between the hips. These joints are like stitched seams. (Similar joints are in the skull, too.) In all of these joints, lots of fine strands of cable and a thin piece of teflon, through which the strands run, fill a small gap between the bones. There is no open space in the joint and no bag surrounding it. There is usually no lubricant either. The strands and teflon that cross the joint hold it tightly closed so that the bones that make up the joint can't move at all.

Why don't these joints move? There are two reasons: The first applies only to women. During the birth of a baby, the child comes through a large hole in the center of the pelvis. All the joints in the pelvis have to give a bit— usually an inch or so—to let the baby out more easily. During the last few months of pregnancy, these joints gradually loosen to let this happen. After the birth, they tighten up again. The other reason is that these joints serve as a "strain relief." If you fall or are hit hard on the pelvis or head, or if your brain wants to grow, these joints usually give way before the bones break. This prevents a fracture in a group of bones where this would be particularly bad. The breaks in the joints are usually incomplete and a few long strands are left to hold the bones together while more cords and teflon filling are made to reconnect the bones.

At the beginning, I mentioned that all types of arthritis, other than the arthritis of aging, are due to problems in the lining of the joints. That's not quite true. There is a problem with the teflon cap itself in the arthritis of aging, which probably is the *result of the changes in the bone lying immediately beneath it.* In addition, there are rather rare types of arthritis where the problem is in the teflon cap itself, which includes those joints that don't move at all. With these exceptions, all types of arthritis, other than wear and tear, really are the result of problems in the joint bag. Some of them seem to be due to problems in the lining itself. Others involve the blood vessels in the lining. In general, the basic problem *isn't in the bone or teflon cap themselves.*

One thing you must be careful of in identifying or treating arthritis is the look-alikes. There are a lot of illnesses that look or feel like arthritis but really aren't. Throughout this book are some sections on the look-alikes, which are listed in the index. If you have doubts about your diagnosis, if you're trying to decide for yourself what's wrong with you, or if things aren't going well with the usual treatments, take a glance at these sections. Perhaps the disease you have isn't arthritis at all, or it isn't the type you originally thought it was. It can make a real difference in the treatment.

Before you continue there are two simple, but important things I want to mention. First, Teflon® is a trademark of E. I. DuPont, Inc. for their patented fluorocarbon polymers.

The term *teflon* is used in this book to refer to the material called cartilage because of some similar properties between the two. It does not mean that our joints normally have Teflon® in them, or that there is any relationship between DuPont and our joints. In short, "Teflon®" and "teflon" don't mean the same thing at all.

Second, most of the treatments in this book involve the use of either devices or drugs that are only available by doctor's prescription. The government, through the FDA, has wisely restricted the use of these items in this way. Although these treatments have helped many people, all of them have their side effects and dangers. Some are minimal, a few are very serious. And not all work for everyone. The medical care of your arthritis, if you choose to see a physician for it, is something you and your doctor must map out on an individual basis. The information in this book is to let you know what's available at this time. It isn't and can't be a plan or direct recommendation of medical care for you. The information isn't a recommendation to use drugs and devices for purposes not authorized by the FDA, or obtained through illegal means.

2

Wear and tear arthritis

THE ARTHRITIS OF AGING is the result of wear and tear. It usually happens in people over fifty, or in joints that have been damaged. The damage can be caused by an old injury or some other type of arthritis. The arthritis of aging doesn't usually happen in people under fifty, although a few people do get it before this age. Those who do get it are very susceptible to this type of arthritis. If they do much work using some of their joints over and over it can cause the bones to age prematurely. Then the arthritis of aging sets in at age thirty or forty.

This wear and tear type of arthritis is due to improper repair of the *tiny hairline fractures that appear in the bones with normal activity.* The poor repair then causes the joints to age faster than they should. For this reason, wear arthritis, or *osteoarthritis* as it's called by doctors, occurs in joints at the ends of bones that work a lot. The last two joints on the fingers, the knees, hips, and back are those which are usually hit by this problem. Wear arthritis has several typical features: the joints I just mentioned are hurt with use, and are often restricted in how far you can bend them. Sudden attacks of pain and swelling can occur and the joint can turn red with these as well. The swelling may happen with very little pain. These sudden attacks aren't necessarily related to your use of the joint. *All types of arthritis hurt more when a joint hasn't been used for a while, and all types feel better after the joint is worked about gently.* In wear arthritis, the ends of the bones near the joints often thicken with little hard nodules or lumps of bones that stick up. This is particularly easy to see at the ends of bones in the fingers.

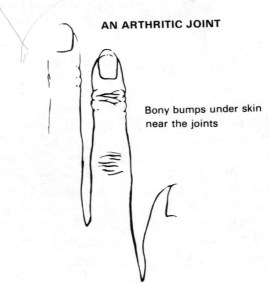

AN ARTHRITIC JOINT

Bony bumps under skin
near the joints

Let's discuss the reasons arthritis of aging develops and what happens along the way. You'll see why the pain and sudden swelling occur, why it aches when you first start to move, why you can't bend the joints as far as you'd like, and what to do about it. There are also several diseases that look like wear arthritis, but have completely different treatments. Be sure to look carefully at the section at the end of this chapter, since mistakes are easy to make and are important to catch.

Almost all the joints that get wear arthritis are "rolling block" joints, that have large, flattened surfaces that roll against each other. The surfaces are made out of a Teflon®-like material that absorbs lubricant onto itself, and is replaced from the bone below as it gradually wears away at the surface. The arthritis of aging is not due to a problem in the teflon. Instead *the problem is in the bone itself*. The bone under the joint absorbs the weight on the joints as they move. Anything that "absorbs" a weight can't work like a sponge. It has to transfer that weight immediately to something else. It can distribute where it puts the weight, but there can be no delay in the transfer. It's like a heavy truck going down a road. The road surface absorbs the weight (downward force) from the tires, but the roadbed, under the pavement, still gets all the weight of the truck. The weight is distributed so that the tires don't cut holes and ruts, but if the roadbed isn't good, the pavement above will crack and the road will eventually be destroyed. With the joints, the cap transfers the force or weight to the bone immediately below. From the pressure of this weight this bone generates an electrical force to tell the controllers where to strengthen it. The network of marble and fibers in the bone often cracks a little. These cracked spots lose their electrical force, and chemicals are released that cause small parts of the bone to be broken down and replaced. The new framework isn't always well made, and what should be a strong and regular network is put up crooked and won't hold the strain. If it breaks easily under the next load, the poorly repaired area must again be repaired and so on. With each repair the mistakes are multiplied. The botched-up repairs in the bones cause some weakening and thinning of the bones at the ends, but there is still enough strength for them to support their loads. The problem is at the joint surface. The teflon is made by things similar to the controllers in the bones. These controllers sense how much teflon to produce for the cap on the joint from the electrical forces of the bone underneath them. There's nothing in the joint itself telling them what to do. The less crystal-like this bone is, the weaker the force is. After a period of years of poor repair, the electrical force the teflon controllers feel is weak. As a result, they make a teflon cap that is thin and wears through easily. Remember, there's nothing from the joint itself to tell them what to do.

This thin cap raises two problems. First, there is less cushion to carry the weight and force across the joint to the bone on the other side. Tiny fractures appear in the bones across the joint even more easily. Second, it's the cap that actually lubricates the joint. The lubrication fluid is made by the lining of the joint, but the actual lubrication comes from the fluid retained in the cap and forced out as the joint moves. The thin cap holds less fluid, and can release only a small portion of what it should when the joint moves. The caps rub, wear fast, and the bones under the caps hurt: The joint feels stiff when you start to move as well as later, after the joint has been used for some time.

The pain from the arthritis of wear comes from two sources. The first is the bone itself. (This is the only type of arthritis where the pain actually does come from the bone.) The reason is linked to the breakdown of bone structure below the joints. When the bone network needs remodeling, chemical signals are released to soften the marble and get the controllers to remove it. These chemicals also cause the nerves to carry a signal of pain up to the brain. Usually the day-to-day remodeling doesn't seem painful to us because the amount of chemicals released is so small that the nerves don't usually sense their presence. With wear arthritis, so much bone is removed and so much remodeling done that these chemicals are released in large quantities, causing pain. The ends of the bones *under the joint* really do hurt. These same chemicals are also released into the joint as the teflon caps rub against the lining. When the chemicals reach the lining, they cause pain to be felt from the joint itself. The lining also produces more fluid, in an effort to better lubricate the area. Sometimes so much fluid is made that the joint bag swells. The chemicals causing all this are called *prostaglandins,* or P-G's for short.

The P-G's also seem to be involved in another aspect of wear and tear arthritis. More bone than usual is constantly being made at the ends near the joint. Some of this bone, though, is made in areas where no pressure or force is transferred at all!

How can this be when bone is laid down according to the electrical forces, which are only within the bone? There is another thing that causes the bones to be laid down: the P-G's. They leak out from the bone at the edges of the joints, and *along their lines of leakage, cause new bone to form. This can happen at any site in the body where leakage occurs.* The leakage of this material from the base of the joint causes the growths of new bone that tend to surround the joint. This can be a serious problem with the back. The joints in the back are a flexible hinge type, and there is no "free space" in the joint for the P-G's to leak. As a result they immediately come out around the joint, and cause new bone to form up alongside it. In the back, this can really limit how far the bones can bend. The new bone that forms where no bone should be at all are *spurs.* As the spurs strike each other or normal bone, they too fracture, often at a microscopic level. This releases more P-G's, which reach nearby nerves, causing more pain, more problems.

FORMATION OF SPURS

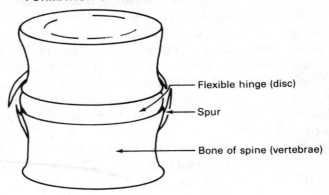

Flexible hinge (disc)

Spur

Bone of spine (vertebrae)

As the teflon cap thins, it actually wears through in spots. When this happens, bare bone is exposed to wear in the joint. As the joint moves, some of this bone breaks off, leaving fragments the size of fine sand. Two problems arise. The first is that the bones simply grind away. The second centers around the joint scavenger cells. The scavenger cells are in the lining to pick up tiny flakes of joint cap that come off. These flakes, when teflon, are not crystals, and the scavengers remove them without any special problem. The fragments of bone, however, are a mineral crystal. Although they must still be removed to protect the joint, this crystal activates the scavengers, which release P-G's and other chemicals. These cause the pain, swelling, and redness that can happen suddenly in both wear arthritis and other kinds where crystals are in the joint. The bits of bone then cause a second crystal-induced arthritis that can be very painful. This crystal arthritis usually hits one joint at a time, and comes on very suddenly, sometimes in minutes. The crystals might have been there for some time, but it's only after they are picked up that they cause arthritis. If they just sit in the joint and rub around, they can damage the cap, but won't cause pain.

This crystal arthritis can be caused by almost any type of crystal. It's the cause of the arthritis of gout and several other diseases. One particular type of bone crystal, *calcium pyrophosphate* is the cause of a disease very similar to gout in the type of joint pain it causes, called *pseudogout*. It usually goes along with wear arthritis, but can be a part of other diseases as well. Stressful situations, such as a heart attack or operations, seem to bring about the scavenging of these crystals, leading to sudden arthritis. Other crystals including crystals of cortisone-like drugs that had been injected into the joint as a treatment for arthritis can also cause the problem.

Wear arthritis in the hip is somewhat different from wear arthritis in other joints. The hip is a ball and socket joint. The weight of the body is distributed over a large area, and the strain on the joint is small compared to the knee and fingers. Why does the hip get wear arthritis? Sometimes the joint is small and poorly formed from birth. Occasionally, an infection or childhood rheumatoid arthritis is the start of it. Usually the answer is blood. Most joints and bones get blood from several arteries and if one closes off, blood is brought in from other routes. The hip in many people is a bit different. It has a few or sometimes only one artery carrying blood into the joint. If one of those arteries closes off, even partially, the bone under the joint can lose most of its blood supply. The controllers then can't get the materials needed to make more marble and rope, nor can they carry out their job of directing where things go. At worst, they die. The bone then cracks easily below the joint and poor repairs, or none at all, are made. The teflon cap becomes thin, due to loss of electrical force under the cap, and it soon simply wears away. So, wear arthritis of the hip is basically a blood supply problem.

Why does this happen? The main reason is smoking, especially cigarettes. Smoking gradually closes off the arteries throughout the body. This is especially true for people whose arteries to the hip were small from birth, or who have fewer arteries than usual; the blood supply runs short, and the bone underlying the joint literally dies. So if you don't want arthritis of the hip, don't smoke. If you already have the arthritis, be sure to stop smoking right away before the entire hip is destroyed.

In the back, wear arthritis poses a different problem, related to how the back works. The back is a series of bones connected by a series of flexible hinges which allow the back to bend in all directions and to twist. The "back" bone actually runs up and down the center of the body and is really a central support pillar. From the rear of the blocks of bone come rings, again made of bone. Going down the middle of these rings is the important stuff. From the base of the head to the bottom of the chest is a thick cable of nerves, like a large telephone cable. The nerves in this cable carry messages from the brain to the rest of the body to tell the body what to do and when. They also carry messages from the body to the brain to tell it what's going on. Between each pair of rings two smaller cables come off the main one and travel to each side. These cables, though much smaller, have thousands of wires in them carrying electrical signals. Even after the main cable—the spinal cord—stops, these small cables keep coming off and go down to the tailbone. These cables have amplifiers to "boost" the signal along the way, about every quarter-inch. If the cable is pinched, the amplifiers are in trouble and send out static. The pinching causes extra signals to go to the brain and down the nerve in the other direction as well. The pinching translates into pain (a wrong signal) and weakness and loss of feeling (amplifiers so badly damaged they don't send any message at all).

You might think that the biggest problem in arthritis of the back is from the flexible joints wearing out. To a limited extent, this does happen in some people, but it isn't necessarily related to any arthritis elsewhere. These joints, called discs, are made in two parts. The inner one is a springy, rubbery material like silicone rubber or a ball of rubber bands. It's surrounded by a tough plastic coating that is glued to the bones above and below. The discs are well-equipped to repair themselves throughout life, but occasionally two problems develop. The first is that the inner, rubbery material may become less springy, and shrinks a bit. This doesn't usually cause much trouble in its own right. However, if the *outer layer of the disc weakens,* the inner rubber may bulge outward. If the bulge goes up or down, the bones seal it off. If it goes to the front, there's nothing there for it to hit that can't move aside. However, if the bulge goes to the rear, it can hit one

ARTHRITIS IN THE SPINE

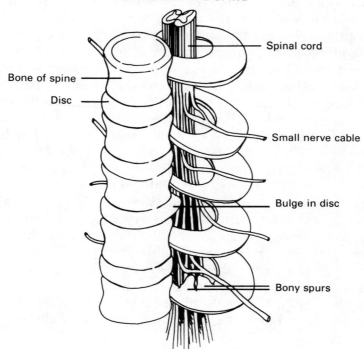

Spinal cord

Bone of spine

Disc

Small nerve cable

Bulge in disc

Bony spurs

or several of the nerves, causing pain and stopping them from working. Other things, besides aging of the disc, cause this bulging. It occurs in young as well as old people. In either case, the weakening or bulging of the disc causes problems only by pinching the nerve. For that reason disc problems traditionally have been considered a nerve problem rather than an arthritic one. For that reason, disc problems are not discussed much in this book.

The main problem from wear arthritis in the spine is that lots of spurs form. These usually grow out along the line of the flexible hinge that joins the bones. As these grow out, they can grow so far as to pinch or hit the nerves. This can cause pain, and may seem to be a "disc" problem. Down low in the spine, these spurs sometimes become so large that they narrow off the tube through which the cables travel (the spinal canal). If the narrowing is serious enough, the nerves can be injured.

In the neck area, the rings of bones form true joints. As these joints form spurs, they can also trap the nerves and pinch them. But, since these joints are similar to those in our hands, the joints here can give a typical arthritic pain, but *only in the neck*. The pain is always directly in the back of the neck, off center just a bit. It's worse when bending the head forward and turning. Like arthritis elsewhere, gentle use eases the pain after a while.

Usually arthritic pain is something you can actually feel in the joint. Occasionally it feels like it comes from the ends of the bone near the joint. When the pain is due to a nerve being pinched, it's completely different. Nerves are like a telephone cable. The brain is at one end and at the other is whatever the nerve cable goes to. If the cable is damaged, the brain thinks the problem is at the place where the cable goes to. It doesn't think the problem is in the cable itself. It's like a phone line cut between you and someone else. When the line is cut, you think the problem is with the other person's phone, not the cable between phones. When a spur, or disc, hits a nerve coming out from the spine, the pain that you feel will seem to come from wherever the nerve goes.

Let's summarize a few things about wear arthritis before discussing what to do about it.

The Characteristics of Wear Arthritis

Involves the fingers' last two joints, knees, hips, back, and neck. Usually occurs in people over 40, but may occur in any joint previously damaged.

Joints hurt and swell on and off. The joint may enlarge without actually swelling because of the growth of bone around the joint.

Limits how much you can move the joint. Some stiffness when first starting to move can be worked away. Pain, stiffness, and grating of the joints increase after more use.

What Causes It?

Poor repair of the bone under the joint with loss of electrical force and deterioration of the teflon.

Formation of spurs.

Poor blood supply in the hip.

Flakes of bone breaking off into the joint.

What Can You Do About It?

When it comes to treating arthritis, be careful. There is a lot of junk around. Fad diets, medicines, vitamins, lotions, rub-in linaments, and the like. Almost all of them are junk. There are no cures, but there are some really good treatments that work to fight the pain and the worsening of the disease. *The treatments that do help work because they go to the basics of why things go wrong.*

The first thing to forget about is most diets for arthritis. None of them have anything that can help you. The same is true of vitamins for arthritis, including ones marketed especially for this problem. Among the vitamins, be very careful to avoid preparations with lots of A, D, E, and C, since these can do harm. Stay away from mineral supplements since they can't help and some can hurt badly. Most of the mineral supplements that were terribly bad have been banned by the FDA. But be careful not to take added magnesium, iodine, potassium, or fluoride, unless there is some other special medical reason for doing so. There is a special treatment for softening of the bones, which involves using calcium, vitamin D, and sometimes fluoride as well as female hormones. This disease is not a form of arthritis and the treatment is usually bad for arthritis if there is no softening of the bones present as well.

An average diet is all that's needed. If you want to take a vitamin, choose the "one a day" type, either by the Miles Laboratories, or any generic once-daily vitamin equal to it. All these provide the vitamins and minerals in 100% of the "RDA" but no more. Don't take added vitamin C. Vitamin deficiencies don't cause arthritis, and *your arthritis is not due to a lack of vitamins.* Added vitamins can't help and can do much harm.

What will help? On the long range, stop smoking if you're doing that now. I can't stress too much how important circulation is in the tiny blood vessels, and how badly smoking impairs it. You can't see directly or feel what's happening until your joints, particularly the hip, are permanently damaged. If you already have the damage, stop smoking or the arthritis at the hip will progress at a rapid rate. The smoking problem applies strongest to the arthritis of the hip. It may make less of a difference at the other joints.

The next thing is *proper exercise.* Improper exercise is a veritable disaster to the joints. Complete lack of exercise isn't good either, since the joints rely on exercise to know when to make their lubricant. Any type of exercise that will subject the joints to sudden pressures is bad. The joints lubricate and cushion themselves best when a gradual but strong pressure is put on them. Sudden pressure puts too much weight on the teflon caps all at once, and the fluid can't be released from the cap fast enough to lubricate properly. In addition, the sudden pressure is cushioned poorly and fractures the bone under the caps. These small cracks only cause more of the poor remodeling to take place. The poor remodeling, in its turn, causes poor teflon formation. So the arthritis is just worsened by these kinds of exercises. In addition, the sudden pressure squeezes the P-G's we talked about out of the cap and into the bone surrounding the joint. This causes more spurs to form, and the ones that are there to enlarge. *So don't use running, skiing, jumping, jogging, tennis, racquetball as types of sports.* This is true whether you have an old knee injury and want to avoid wear arthritis from developing in the first place, or if you have arthritis already and want to avoid its progressing.

Sports that put a steady but slow and smooth pressure and strain on the joints are good. For example, *swimming, bicycling, and moderate weight lifting are all good.* These apply a steady pressure, allowing the joints to lubricate properly during use, thus avoiding the formation of new fractures, while the joints preserve their function.

What about less active exercises? For the fingers and hands, a simple squeezing motion is best. It's easy to do this with a small ball, like a tennis ball or smaller. Hold it in the palm of your hand, with the palm facing up. Slowly but strongly tighten your fist around the ball and then relax. Let the whole tightening and relaxing cycle take about 5-10 seconds. Do it slowly, but with as much strength as you can muster without much pain. Then put the ball down. This next part without the ball is very important to retain full use of your hand. Open and close your fist slowly but close it as fully as you can. You may not be able to get it into a full fist or completely closed, but do it as far as you can. If you find it very painful, it'll be more comfortable to do these exercises with your hand under warm water. Do the exercises a minimum of ten times each. If time and comfort permit, work up to 50 times with and without the ball with each hand, but don't start at 50 times. The best way to do all these exercises, including all that follow, is to *exercise for about 10 minutes four to six times a day.* Don't try to do the whole day's exercises at one sitting. Start with only a few repeats, and gradually work up. The real key to using the exercises is to do them several times a day at the minimum. The signals that the teflon caps and joint lining get from the first set of exercises tells them how much lubricant and new teflon to make over the next 12 hours or so, not for the whole next week. Your joints need a constant, gentle reminder of how much lubricant and teflon to make. A single hard kick will only tell them to swell up, nothing more.

For the wrists: Lightly hold the ball in your hand. Slowly, while gently squeezing the ball, bend the wrist up and down, with your palm facing down. Again, start at 5 times each hand for 4 sessions or more a day. Work up to fifty. If the wrist gets sore at first, do it under warm water.

For the knees, take the exercises easy at first. Sit so that your feet clear the floor, like on the edge of a table. Slowly straighten your leg as far as you can go. Hold the leg up for a second or so. Let it drop down slowly. Then pull it back as far as you can, so that it doubles up if possible. Start with this exercise about 10 times a session. Don't try to do a whole day's exercises at once. After you're up to about 40 times per session by making gradual increases, gently start trying knee bends. Go down as far as you can with comfort, and then up again. Use a chair to partially support your weight and help yourself at first. Don't replace your earlier exercises with these. Add a few on at the end of each session. Work gradually to 10 of these several times a day, added on at the end of each session. Go down just as far as is comfortable. *Remember that repeating the exercises several times a day is more important than the number you do at one session.* If you're really fat, or if your knees are in terrible shape, check for advice before doing the knee bends.

For the shoulder and hip: If your arthritis involves these joints, the exercises are somewhat different. Here the joint naturally has a wide range of motion. The exercises are designed to restore and keep this range. For the shoulder, start with your arm out across your chest. Slowly swing it around as far back as you can. Then go from back to front over your head and down again. As with the other exercises, start with groups of four, repeated several times a day. If possible increase to 20 or more a session. As your shoulder becomes limber, you'll be able to put a small weight, like a paperweight, in your hand for added strain on the shoulder. The exercise for the hip is very similar. Stretch your leg out in front and all the way up, so it's as near level with the floor as you can make it. Take it across your body too to the opposite side. Starting from here, swing the leg in front of you around to the back as far as you can. When you get to the rear, or as far to the rear as you can, let the leg drop down. Carry it through with that motion to the front and start again. Start with 4 repeats and work up to 20. Knee bends are good hip exercises as well. With the exercises for the hips and shoulders, if you are likely to dislocate the joint (you'll know from past experience) avoid getting the arm and leg in a position where this can happen.

I know of no special exercises of use for arthritis of the back.

Remember that with all these exercises, frequent repetition is the key. You don't need to force your joints to work as hard as you can, but you do need to work them often.

This will keep you limber but what do you do about the pain? Is there any medicine you can take to help prevent the arthritis from progressing and becoming more painful yet? That question brings me to the next big topic: the medications used to treat arthritis of aging. The central thing to understand is that *all medicines work by doing something chemically to the body.* Usually the chemicals work for only a short while—a few hours, a day or so. None produce a permanent change. Once the drug or chemical is gone, things go back to what they were. *The only exception to this is the antibiotics.* These drugs are not there to alter the body's chemistry at all. They selectively poison the bugs causing the infection, and avoid interfering in the body's own chemistry.

For wear arthritis, and for many other types as well, the main family of drugs affect the P-G's. As you remember, these are the main chemicals causing the pain of arthritis, the growth of bony spurs, and the removal of bone as well. There are many drugs that lower P-G production. Differences are only ones of patent rights. Since there are so many of these drugs, and they are similar, I'll only explore the most useful.

The cheapest of the group is aspirin. It also is the fastest-working but not the most effective. Usually two or three tablets (5 grain size) must be taken every 6 to 8 hours on an ongoing basis. Aspirin is upsetting to many people's stomachs, however, especially in that quantity day after day. This can cause stomach and intestinal ulcers. In addition, particularly in people over 60, it has bad effects on the ears and brain that limit its use, causing dizziness, loss of hearing, and confusion. Use one of the buffered aspirin—the generic, Bufferin®, AlkaSeltzer®, Ascriptin®, delayed release forms (Ecotrin®)—or use antacids with the aspirin to get around the stomach irritation problem. Many people prefer one of the new prescription "replacements" for aspirin. These drugs are not similar to Tylenol® or codeine. Tylenol® and its generic equivalents (acetaminophen) should not be used for arthritis, since it is damaging to the liver with repeated use. It also is not very effective for arthritic pains. The replacement for aspirin that is substantially better than the others is Clinoril®. It comes in sizes of 150 and 200 mg. Some people with wear arthritis need as little as 150 mg (1 tablet) a day. Others need as much as two 200 mg tablets (or occasionally three) twice a day. While taken only twice daily, instead of 4-6 times, this medicine is actually more effective than aspirin for the pain and swelling, and far less likely to upset the stomach. If it does cause stomach upset, use an antacid (I recommend Titralac®) or a new drug for ulcers (Tagamet®) along with it. The main problem with Clinoril® is that a few people develop diarrhea. Sometimes this clears up on its own, sometimes added treatment is needed. Usually the Clinoril® is enough help to make the added problem worth putting up with. If not, alternatives are discussed in the last chapter. If the pain and stiffness aren't satisfactorily controlled with Clinoril®, the next drug to try is Indocin®, which is a close chemical cousin to Clinoril®. The dosage is between 25 and 50 mg three times a day. Problems are more common with this drug, however, than with Clinoril®, particularly stomach irritation.

What if you're allergic to aspirin? First, an upset stomach from aspirin is not an allergy—it is a direct irritation. Try the aspirin or Clinoril® with both antacids and Tagamet® if needed. Why keep trying if your stomach's upset? You won't find any drugs that work better, so give them as much of a chance as you can. Aspirin allergy is a special thing—hives and wheezing (asthma) from taking aspirin. If you have asthma, or asthma plus nasal polyps, that alone doesn't mean you are allergic to aspirin. Indeed, many people who have asthma, with or without the polyps, are helped by aspirin. If you really do have an aspirin allergy, don't try either aspirin or any of the aspirin-like drugs. Try *salicylic acid* (Arthropan®, Disalid®, Magan®, Trilisate®). This is also less upsetting to the stomach than aspirin, and may help if both aspirin and Clinoril® irritate the stomach too much. It doesn't usually work as well as either of these but, unlike Tylenol®, it is safe for long-term use.

What about cortisone? It will work for the pain of wear arthritis. In fact, much of what it does is identical to aspirin and Clinoril®: it decreases the production of the P-G's. It will, however, cause your bones to lose their marble and weaken. As this goes on in the bone under the joint, it will make the arthritis progress all the more. Cortisone can be injected into a joint now and then, but when it's put into the joint, it can diffuse (migrate slowly) into the bone under it, and cause the same problem. How often can you get coristone injections for wear arthritis safely? Never when the injection is into a muscle, like with the arm or hip. Never if it's tablets. On rare occasion only into a joint directly: but preferably not more than once a year into only one joint in the whole body. The same problems apply to all the synthetic forms of cortisone, as well. The last chapter has a longer discussion of the use of coristone in arthritis and its problems, if you're interested.

In order to work well, medicines like aspirin, Clinoril®, and salicylic must be taken on a daily basis, although the amount may vary according to how bad the arthritis is. All of them require 1-4 days before they really start to work. An on-again, off-again way of taking them doesn't work nearly as well. When wear arthritis flares up just once in a while, occasional use is fine. This is very rare. If arthritis is present all the time, but only hurts some of the time, it is much better to take at least some of the medicine all the time. This prevents the flair ups, and probably will help prevent progression of the disease.

When the pain does flair up resting the joint and applying heat helps temporarily. Pain relievers that don't affect the P-G's work quickly for limited relief. Tylenol®, acetaminophen, is OK in a small dosage. In general, don't use it more than an average of 1-2 days a week. Remember, a large number of these medicines and pain relievers, including Nebs®, Empirin®, Excedrin®, have this ingredient in them. These latter two contain phenacetin, a drug similar to Tylenol®, which may cause severe kidney damage.* Our body also makes it into Tylenol®. Then there are the narcotics. The mildest of them are propoxyphene (Darvon, Dolene®) and codeine. There are stronger ones as well, including Talwin®, Demerol® (meperidine), Dilaudid®, LevoDromoran®, and Methadone®, all of which are estremely effective for pain in pill form, but only for temporary use in arthritis. Highly addictive, they all cause constipation, nausea, sleepiness or excitation, and occasionally hallucinations. All the medicines in this group are only for brief use when the pain simply can't be controlled by Clinoril® and similar drugs alone. None have the danger from long-term use that Tylenol® has, but be careful about this. Most of them are also sold in combination with acetaminophen. Don't use this form of the drug. In general, Darvon®, codeine, and Talwin® have the least addicting potential and are the most suitable for use. Talwin® is the most potent of the three.

---

*Although these potential problems with Tylenol® and phenacetin make them relatively undesirable for continuous, long-term use, these drugs do appear safe when used 3-4 times a day, for as long as a few weeks time. Tylenol® is substantially less effective for pain than aspirin or phenacetin, and often must be used near the maximum safe dosage. For an average-sized adult, this maximum is 1,000 mg (3 tablets or 2 extra-strength pills) every 6 hours.

If you're wondering about the "over the counter" preparations and drugs you can buy without prescription, that are advertised on TV, or in magazines, take a look at the end of the last chapter for the full story. The short version of that story is simple: forget them.

Are there any medications or treatments that halt the progress of wear arthritis? This question doesn't have a clear answer right now. For sure, there is no special diet or group of exercises, other than avoiding additional damage to the joints, that offers any hope. Although the FDA won't permit aspirin, Clinoril® and similar drugs to be advertised for the prevention of arthritis pending more evidence, you should remember that only these drugs get at the basis of what causes the spurs to form and what increases the poor repair of the bone underlying the joint. There is every reason to think that *these drugs do slow the worsening of wear arthritis.* In order to do this, they must be taken every day without fail. How much is needed? Right now there's no clear answer to this. But we do know that when aspirin is used to prevent other things like hardening of the arteries and blood clots the dose is small. Probably 2 or 3 aspirin a day, or 150 mg of Clinoril® is enough. Salicylate may not be effective for this, though.

What if the joints are just shot? For some of them there is a replacement. Remember that these replacements are not perfect. In fact, some of them are pretty poor compared to the real thing. If no use is left in the joints or, in the case of the hip only, if the pain is very severe, the replacements are worth it. The ones for the hip and, to a lesser extent, the knee are fairly good. The replacements last 7-10 years; 1-5% of these people have real problems with infections in the replaced joints. Another several percent get blood clots from them. But 80-90% of people who have the replacements are able to walk again, which makes them worthwhile. If you are overweight almost all doctors who do the replacements will require you to lose weight first. For the fingers, toes, and elbows, another type of joint replacement is available. It is a rubber shaft or column with a flair in the middle that acts as a pad. This joint is put in between two bones. It pads them, and keeps them in line while they bend against one another. Infections aren't as much a problem with these, but they do wear out.

The spurs that form in wear arthritis pose a problem if they begin to hit nerves or become so large that the bones are locked into place. Aspirin and Clinoril® show some promise in preventing or slowing the growth of the spurs. A different approach, used in addition to this, is also available. Remember that the spurs are made by bone marble being laid down where there was previously none. A new drug, Didronel®, can prevent this from happening and can slow the rate of growth of the spurs. The proper amount to use isn't clear for each case at this time, but the growth of the spurs can be measured with a test called a technecium scan. The dosage of Didronel® can be adjusted accordingly. Since too much drug can cause other serious problems, great care must be used with this treatment, and it shouldn't be used for everyone with spur formation.

When you've read this chapter, remember to turn to the last one for more information on the treatments mentioned, and new ones to come.

Look-Alikes

One of the big problems with wear arthritis is things that look like it, but aren't. Some of these are bone diseases, some of them don't involve the bone or joints at all. Most of them are reasonably common, and are things you must be careful about since these look-alikes have special treatments.

The first is Paget's Disease. Here, the controllers themselves are making a mistake. Although this disease usually starts in the end of a bone, the joint isn't involved. Certain groups of controllers constantly remodel the bone at a very fast rate, and do a terrible job of it. They don't appear to sense the electrical force in the bone well. As a result, the bone itself hurts, especially when you stand or press on it. In addition, the bone becomes thicker and warm. If you think the problem is arthritis but the joint isn't stiff and the bone hurts and is warm or large, the problem is either Paget's disease or something else like bone infection or cancer but not arthritis.

Another look-alike is called "reflex sympathetic dystrophy." That's a long name, which like so many medical terms means little. It occurs when an arm or leg isn't used for some time. As a result, the limb and joints hurt and are tender; the skin turns red or pale, and thins out. All this happens because the controllers are sensing too little an electrical force. There's no pressure on the bone to generate electricity. The controllers then release P-G's that both cause the pain and removal of marble from the bone. The treatment for this is Clinoril® and one of the natural signals our body uses to tell the controllers to make more marble. This is called Calcitonin and is given by injection. The key thing to remember is that this look-alike happens in a limb or around a joint that isn't getting much use at all, and usually involves either an entire hand, foot, or limb. To make things more complicated, the original lack of use can be due to arthritis in the first place.

Nerves are easily pinched or irritated at many spots in the body. The pain that comes from this is often confused with arthritis. There are several ways to keep them straight, but one of them isn't where the pain occurs. First, if weakness is part of the problem, a nerve has to be bad. If the pain isn't in just one spot but seems to go somewhere—from the hip down the leg, from the wrist to the thumb or up the arm—from anywhere to anywhere, it is usually a nerve problem, not arthritis.

The cables that hook the muscles to the bones can cause problems that also are look-alikes for arthritis. These cables can become sore for many reasons, and when they do, they may swell and can be every bit as painful as any arthritis. This causes stiffness as well. Here, the pain will go along the length of the cable, and will be much worse whenever you use the bone and muscle the cable hooks up. Unlike the pain from a nerve problem, this pain is much worse right when you use that bone or muscle, only. Unlike arthritis, the pain is along the entire length of the cable, not in a joint.

The last look-alike hasn't been too common so far, in the United States. When the iron supplements in our food are raised, as they will probably be in the future, it will probably become much more common. In this last disease, the body stores too much iron, which it takes in from the food we eat. As a result, there are liver problems, diabetes, and arthritis from the damage the iron causes. The treatment for this disease is to remove the iron from the body. If this isn't done, the illness is long and fatal. The arthritis that it causes—and this is a true arthritis—is like wear arthritis, except that it happens in the main part of the hand and at the base of the fingers. This is very different from the usual pattern. So if you have arthritis that seems like wear arthritis in these areas, or have diabetes or liver problems along with it, have your doctor look for the iron storage disease, called *hemochromatosis*. It has a very special, and successful treatment.

3

Gout

IF YOU MENTIONED GOUT TO SOMEONE, he would probably think of arthritis, or of pain in the foot. If a person is told he has gout, he usually thinks he has a form of arthritis, and that's all. But that isn't the way things work. *Gout is a disease that is present from birth and affects the entire body, not just the joints.* Obviously, if that's the case, gout isn't basically an arthritis. Gout does include arthritis as part of the problem, but the basic disease and the basic problem are much more extensive than that.

The thing that occurs in gout is very simple. Crystals start forming soon after birth, throughout the entire body. These crystals settle out from the body fluids virtually everywhere. The only place they aren't found is in the brain and nerves. The deposits the crystals form in the kidney, blood vessels, around the tendons (the cables that hook the muscles to the bones) and in the joints cause the damage. In each of these areas the crystal deposits lead to a particular, and serious problem.

Where do these crystals come from? The crystals are made from uric acid. Uric acid can dissolve in the blood and body fluids to a limited extent. Some people produce more uric acid than others, and there is more than can be dissolved in the body fluids. It falls out or precipitates and forms crystals. Most of this uric acid does not come from the diet, but is made internally. Why do some people have too much uric acid? There are several reasons. Usually uric acid is removed from the body by the kidney. A few people with hereditary gout have a kidney that removes less uric acid than most. What their kidney thinks is a normal level of uric acid is actually too high. As a result, they always have too much uric acid in the blood. Since the blood is constantly exchanging its uric acid with that in all the other body fluids, the entire body has too much as well. In most people with gout, however, the kidney is normal or only a little off. The problem is that too much uric acid is made internally.

Why does this happen? To best understand this, I will tell you a bit about why the uric acid is made.

You've probably heard about the "genetic code" and perhaps about DNA as well. In short, each cell in our body has a library of computer tapes on which the information our body needs to stay alive is recorded. A complete library is present in most cells we have. Unlike the usual computer tape, the body uses a string of beads to make the tapes. The beads are then read as letters of an alphabet. As new cells are made, each must have a complete set of tapes and, as a result, the library is duplicated frequently. In addition, when the body uses the tapes to make something, it doesn't use the original, but makes a working copy first. As a result, each cell always needs to have beads around to make either library or working copies of the tapes. Since running out of beads means death, a spare supply is always kept on hand. The beads that aren't needed, and the ones that come from the cleanup after a cell dies, are tossed. But before they are tossed, some are broken up and become uric acid. So, people who overproduce uric acid do so by overproducing the beads from which the genetic tapes are made. Having extra beads around can be handy, but obviously, it can lead to real problems when it causes gout. Again, this over-production is inherited and is present from birth.

The causes of gout and, therefore, gout itself are much more common in men than women.

It takes a long time for the crystals to build up to a level where they cause problems. Over a period of decades, they do form these deposits. They don't cause problems until the deposits are spotted by a "scavenger" white blood cell, which picks them up and starts to collect the crystals. The crystals set up a reaction in the blood cell that causes it to release P-G's and some other chemicals. These cause more white blood cells to collect more crystals and release more P-G's. If the reaction is in the joint, the lining releases a large amount of fluid, and the joint swells and hurts. A similar thing happens in the tendons. The crystals collect between the tendon and its sheath. When enough crystals collect, the white blood cells again try to scavenge them, and again set off the painful reaction. Although the painful tendon problem starts earlier, usually by age 35, the pain is milder and not given much notice. The knee and shoulder tendons are usually the ones affected. Joint swelling comes later, for most.

Unlike the tendon problem, which sometimes is a chronic, nagging pain, as well as sudden attacks, the arthritis in gout is almost always a sudden, painful swelling during the first 5 to 10 years of its occurrences. The big toe is the usual place where gout starts although any joint can be involved. I suspect the reason gout sometimes picks the big toe is that this joint gets the most punishment of any, and is pretty sure to have white blood cells there scavenging teflon flakes much of the time. The pain and swelling not only start suddenly, but worsen quickly. Early on and for the first five years or more, the situation is one of repeated severe attacks, not a continuous or on-going arthritis that gradually gets better or worse. Usually only one joint at a time is involved. Later on, if the gout problem is not treated, the joints are so badly involved that several also have attacks at once. After some years, wear and tear arthritis also sets in, and then the joints hurt all the time. Attacks become more frequent because the wear arthritis keeps more white blood cells around at all times to set off the attacks again.

If the pain isn't in the big toe, it can still be gout. The wrist is the other favored joint, but as I mentioned, it can happen in most any joint of the body. Of course, just because there is an attack in the big toe, it doesn't mean that the problem is gout. Other types of arthritis can have sudden attacks here as well.

When gout is really advanced, large deposits of the crystals can actually break through the skin over or around a joint, or in the ear. Before they break through, they feel like a rubbery, or occasionally pebbly lump under the skin. The material in them is a yellow pasty stuff, not a rock crystal the way salt is. These deposits of crystals build up in the joints, too. Remember, they don't necessarily hurt. That happens only if a white blood cell tries to eat one. But they do press their way into the teflon cap on the joint, and destroy it over a period of years. In other words, the amount of pain you experience from gout does not reflect how much damage is being done.

Although gout can be an unpleasant type of arthritis to have, the damage it does in other parts of the body is usually more serious over a period of years than the arthritis itself. The first place of real concern is the kidney. Two things happen here. The first is painless. Deposits of uric acid crystals form throughout the kidney. Normally, there aren't many scavenger cells in the kidney to eat into these and set off much pain. Gradually, the deposits grow in size and press against the cells that make up the kidney. Over a period of years, there can be a steady loss of kidney functioning in many people with gout. In some, it causes kidney failure.

The second is that uric acid crystals can form in the urine. The kidney is a sort of filter for the blood. After going through many tiny strainers and processing channels, the stuff the body wants to get rid of is passed out as urine. Along with other things, the urine contains a fair amount of uric acid. In the few people who have gout because their kidneys remove too little uric acid, this isn't a problem, since their urine contains less than the usual amount. Most people with gout make too much uric acid to begin with. As a result, they have too much uric acid in their urine as well. Just as in the body's internal fluids, crystals form in the urine, too. Frequently these are called kidney stones, although they aren't always a solid stone. Often a large group of crystals forms a sludge in the kidney. The sludge is then released or shaken loose and comes down like a mud pie before it's dried. Frequently, too, a few uric acid crystals pick up a calcium coating that grows and becomes a "calcium stone." The sludge or stone is very irritating to the tiny tube that goes from the kidney to the bladder and causes it to swell. The swelling completely blocks the flow of urine. The kidney, however, keeps on pumping urine under pressure and the entire tube above that spot balloons up. It's this ballooning of the tube that hurts more than the stone itself. Eventually, the sludge or stone is forced through and the ballooning goes down, and the stone is "passed." Passing a kidney stone is painful, but it's just the beginning of problems. People with gout may have this occur repeatedly. Each blockage can permanently damage the kidney, and causes repeated infection. Both of these cause high blood pressure and kidney failure.

Unless properly treated, gout also causes rapid harden-

ing of the arteries, which is far more serious than anything arthritis can do. This leads to high blood pressure,
heart attacks, strokes, senility, and kidney failure later in

EFFECT OF KIDNEY STONE OR SLUDGE

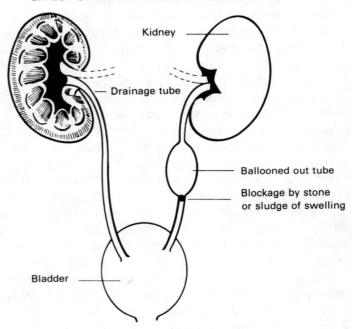

life. If you use the treatments to control the pain of gout
but do not treat the basic disease, this statement is still
true. The treatments for the pain of gout don't control gout
itself, and vice versa. In fact, some of the treatments for
the pain raise the body's level of uric acid, making both
the arthritis and the hardening of the arteries progress
faster than ever unless used without the other type of
treatment, too.

How does gout cause hardening of the arteries? The
story isn't completely clear at this time, but two things
seem critical: The first is a stop-leak system in the blood.

The second is the white blood cells that eat the uric acid crystals. The arteries are tubes that carry blood from the heart and lungs to the entire body. These arteries all have basically the same structure. An elastic covering that stretches and bends with the arteries is on the outside. Under this is a thick layer of muscle. This muscle can make the artery larger or smaller in diameter, letting more or less blood flow, depending on the needs of the part of the body that artery supplies. Under this is more elastic and a tiny bit of muscle. Finally, there is a fine lining. Since the arteries are always bending and stretching, their walls tend to fatigue and form cracks. In addition, occa-

STOP-LEAK SYSTEM IN ARTERY

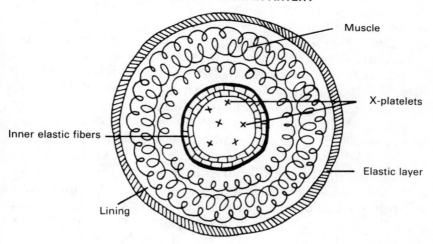

sionally we cut an artery and blood leaks out. For both reasons, a stop-leak system has to be there to prevent these breaks from enlarging and actually letting blood escape.

The stop-leak system is composed of tiny particles, called platelets, that are present in the blood at all times. The lining of the arteries makes a chemical, related to the P-G's, that prevents them from attaching. The platelets themselves, on the other hand, constantly make another chemical (also related to the P-G's) that causes them to attach to the wall of the artery. Ordinarily the lining's chemical is far stronger and prevents the platelets from attaching.

When crystals of uric acid form within the walls of the artery, the situation changes. Scavenger white blood cells are in the blood at all times. These naturally settle out on the walls of the arteries. When they do this, they may come in contact with the crystals of uric acid. As they try to eat one, they immediately set up a reaction similar to the one they start in a joint during a gout attack. However, the reaction is on a much smaller scale. Perhaps a hundredth of an inch of the artery is involved. When the scavenger cells do this, no pain is felt, but they do release chemicals that injure the lining of the artery and chemicals that attract the platelets and make a few of them attach to the damaged area. These few particles that have attached then trigger an avalanche of other platelets onto the wall, causing a clump of platelets to form that is much larger than the original area of irritation that set all this in motion. This clump has tiny muscle-like fibers that pull it together and harden it, so it won't dissolve. These clumps are the things that are hardening of the arteries.

What's so bad about a hundredth of an inch being hurt? All this isn't happening in just one spot. It's happening all over the body, in all the arteries and veins at once. It goes on every day, every hour and it gradually closes the arteries and some of the veins off.

If that's the case, why don't we die immediately from gout? The main reason is that the arteries are much larger than they need to be to carry out their job. It's like having ten-inch water pipes in your house. If you do something that gradually but progressively corrodes them, even the ten-inch pipe will eventually close off. In your body, that means heart attacks, senility, strokes, and kidney failure.

Of course, the more damage there is, the faster it goes. The clump that forms on the damaged area leaves a roughened area on the wall of the artery. This area does cover itself with lining again. But that lining is exposed to the flow of blood which is constantly ripping it off. As the lining is ripped off, the chemicals it was producing to keep the platelets from attaching are not being made. As a result, more platelets constantly attach and that clump continually grows in size. Progressive hardening of the arteries then tends to develop at that spot.

This is why it is important that treatment of gout be directed at the basic process that goes wrong rather than just treating relief of pain.

The Characteristics of Gout

Often the earliest symptom of gout is kidney stones, or sludge, and tendon irritation. Sometimes a large amount of vitamin C will bring out the stones and sludge if they hadn't been present before. The arthritis usually comes later, and always starts out as sudden attacks of pain, redness over the joint, and swelling. The arthritis is much more common in men, and usually starts in the big toe, wrist, knee, or ankle. Frequently, an injury will bring on an attack. The attacks last several days without treatment. Usually at the start, only one joint at a time is affected. Between the attacks the joint is completely normal, at first. After a few years, a premature wear arthritis will begin in the joints involved with gout.

Earlier, I mentioned that there are two parts to the treatment of gout: the treatment of the basic process and the relief of pain. The ideal thing in the treatment is to stop the production of uric acid. If you do this, the body still breaks down the unneeded genetic code beads, but now breaks them down into something that usually won't form crystals and cause the problems uric acid does. The medicine that causes the body to make this change is called *allopurinol* (Zyloprim®), and is ideal for the treatment of gout. *Remember that the medicine doesn't cause any permanent change in how your body handles uric acid, and you must take it daily, every day.* It must be taken whether you have pain or not, whether you feel fine or not. Take it daily, regardless. If you don't, the rest of the problems with gout—the kidney damage, kidney stone formation, and hardening of the arteries—go on. These problems you won't know or feel until it's too late.

Most people can take the *allopurinol* once a day (300 mg, the golden brown colored tablet must be used) to keep their uric acid level within acceptable limits. A few people need to either take a larger amount once a day, or spread it out during the day. Virtually everyone needs at least 300 mg, though.

Changes in diet make very little difference in uric acid levels and gout attacks. Alcohol, however, both raises the amount in the body by preventing the kidney from getting rid of it and makes the uric acid fall out of the blood and form crystals more easily. As mentioned, large amounts of vitamin C (over 250 mg a day) can cause uric acid stones and sludge, and may also raise uric acid levels in the body.

Allopurinol won't relieve an attack of gout, or a kidney stone attack. It's only a prevention for these. To work after attacks of gout have begun takes a while, too. It must lower the blood levels of uric acid for a long enough time to allow the deposits to dissolve. This can take from one to several years, depending on the delay in starting it. In addition, when it is first begun, it can precipitate or bring on an attack of gout, so it's usually wise to either start it slowly (gradually increasing the amount over 1-3 weeks) or use it along with one of the medicines that treat the gout attacks to prevent an attack from starting during the first week or so.

Since *allopurinol* cuts down on the production of uric acid, it will also relieve or prevent the kidney damage and kidney stones that occur with gout. This is the reason that it's better than the other medications available to prevent gout attacks and hardening of the arteries. A few people do need to use something instead of *allopurinol*. The reasons are either a skin rash or liver irritation from the drug. There are two other medicines available: *probenecid* (Benemid®) and *sulfinpyrazone* (Anturane®). Both work by stimulating the kidney to put out more uric acid than normal. The body doesn't try to make up for this loss, so there is a drop in the uric acid level both in the blood and the body as a whole. The level of uric acid in the urine, however, rises and so does the chance of forming kidney stones. So these drugs are not as desirable as *allopurinol*. Like *allopurinol*, both can bring on a gout attack when use is first begun. So they, too, must either be begun gradually, or along with a second drug to prevent a gout attack. The last two drugs can also cause skin rashes. This does not mean a rash will develop as a reaction to the last two of these drugs just because the *allopurinol* caused a rash. Both *probenecid* and *sulfinpyrazone* can upset the stomach, as well.

If you have gout, one of these three must be used: For *probenecid*, the usual minimum dose is one tablet twice daily; for *sulfinpyrazone*, 200 mg twice daily. After a few weeks on any of the three drugs, check your uric acid level to be sure you're taking enough.

What do you do for the pain of gout? If you experience the pain day in and day out, you probably have wear arthritis setting in as a result of repeated gout attacks. Turn to the chapter on this type of arthritis, regarding its treatment. If you have repeated sudden attacks of gout, the best of the current treatments is Clinoril®. If you are taking it to prevent an attack (for example, when starting *allopurinol* or until it has had enough time to work) usually 200 mg twice a day is enough. To treat an acute, recent attack, use 400-600 mg immediately, with antacid and repeat this every 12 hours until the attack is relieved. In general, it takes as long to relieve the attack as the time you waited to start the medicine plus 6-8 hours. If you need faster relief, Indocin® (a relative of Clinoril®) can be used as 50-75 mg on the first dose and 50 mg every 8 hours after. Fastest-working still is *phenylbutazone,* taken as 400 mg on the first dose, and 100 mg every 6 hours. Why not use these last two? Both are extremely irritating to the stomach, and *phenylbutazone,* with repeated use, has many severe reactions. Since you can gain only an added hour or two at the most in your relief, the added risks are not worth taking, except in very unusual instances. If used, Indocin® and especially *phenylbutazone* must always be taken with a liquid antacid.

An old treatment for gout attacks is *colchicine.* When injected into the vein, it works about as fast as Clinoril® or even faster, and has few bad effects. This isn't a convenient way to take your medicine, however. Colchicine tablets, when used to treat a gout attack, work quite slowly and always cause diarrhea and cramping before you're through. They are not recommended for gout attacks, except for use by people with true aspirin allergies, who also should not use Clinoril® (see index). One or two tablets taken every few hours until some balance is reached between joint and stomach troubles is advised. To prevent a gout attack, 1 tablet 2-3 times a day is often enough, and is useful when starting the "curative" drugs discussed earlier. A combination with Benemid® (ColBenemid®) is available on the market.

Cortisone-like drugs, such as *prednisone* or Decadron® will work for gout, but not reliably whether used in pill form or joint injection. *Cortisone and related drugs are not recommended for gout.*

If you treat gout promptly and properly, special exercises are not needed. If your joints hurt all the time, you'd better assume some second type of arthritis is taking place as well, often of the wear and tear variety.

What about the hardening of the arteries? If you start treating the gout condition early enough by using one of the three "prevention" drugs, *allopurinol, probenecid,* or *sulfinpyrazone,* within a few years of onset of either kidney stones or joint attacks, probably no other treatment is needed. If you didn't treat it properly, however, or if gout was discovered after age 40, additional treatments to slow the rate of hardening of the arteries are desirable. The intensity with which you should treat this depends on several other things. The first is whether or not you smoke. Smoking causes hardening of the arteries to progress much more rapidly than otherwise. If you smoke and have gout, a much more intensive treatment is needed. There is a material, called HDL (high density lipoprotein), in the blood that *protects* against hardening of the arteries. If you have little of this material (below 45mg%) then more intensive treatment is needed.

What are these treatments? One type involves drugs that raise the HDL level, our natural protection against hardening of the arteries. So far, only limited success has been had along these lines using the drugs, Lorelco® and Atromid®. Only a few people have an increase in this material so its success from person to person is unpredictable. All the other treatments, which don't vary in effectiveness, involve the *platelets.* They all cut down on the ease with which the platelets attach to the walls of the arteries. The main drug for this purpose is aspirin (buffered aspirin or Bufferin® will also do, but not Tylenol®). For people with gout who don't smoke and have a reasonable HDL level, one aspirin a day is probably all that's needed, along with the usual treatments for gout. If you either smoke or have a low HDL level, then additional treatments are needed. If the HDL level is under 40,

Lorelco® or Atromid® are worth a try to see if they will increase this level. If not, or if you smoke, then the next additional treatment to use is *sulfinpyrazone* (yes, the same drug mentioned before) at 200 mg four times a day to both lower the uric acid and work against the platelets. If this poses a problem in regard to kidney stones, an alternative is to use the gout treatment recommended earlier in this chapter, and add in Persantine® 1 tablet four times a day. According to the situation, several other drugs that work on the platelets may also be useful: Periactin®, Optimine®, and Clinoril®. Remember, though, that all these "additional" drugs to prevent hardening of the arteries are additional to aspirin, which is really the most effective drug for this purpose.

This may seem like too much fuss over hardening of the arteries. Remember, gout plus other things, like smoking or a low HDL level, spell real trouble and death in the long run. The effort is well spent to prevent what will certainly happen if you "leave well enough alone."

There are a few other things worth mentioning about gout. The first is that the diagnosis of gout isn't always easy. If it's in the family that can be a clue. The first thing to go wrong isn't always a pain in the big toe, however. In many people, pain in the tendons comes first, primarily at the knee and shoulder. A blood test for the uric acid level is used most of the time for diagnostic purposes, though there are several problems with this test. The first is that a high uric acid level doesn't always mean gout. The usual, cheap test isn't very accurate. There are many other things in the blood that "look" like uric acid in this test, but aren't. So if your uric acid level is borderline, or if it's high and you think the problem may not be gout, a more refined method must be used: the uricase method for uric acid.

Another confusing thing is that during a gout attack, the blood level of uric acid may be normal and remain so for a few days. A normal uric acid level by either method during a sudden attack of arthritis doesn't mean it isn't gout. To make things even more confusing, several other types of arthritis can cause sudden attacks that look and feel just like gout. To settle the matter, fluid sometimes has to be taken from the swollen joint and examined under a microscope for uric acid crystals. That usually gives a definite answer.

A number of drugs used for high blood pressure and heart disease, called diuretics, raise the uric acid level. All diuretics do this except Selacryn®, which is not available now. This high level of uric acid results from the ability of these drugs to stop the kidney from removing uric acid from the body. This, of course, is one of the ways gout occurs naturally as well. A high uric acid level from this cause is of as much concern as if it were from natural gout, even if no joint pain occurs. The reason is that the effect of the uric acid on the progression of hardening of the arteries remains the same. Since these diuretics are usually used in conditions where hardening of the arteries is already a problem, adding anything to cause this to worsen isn't a good idea. Because of their ability to lower the uric acid level in the blood while working as a diuretic, drugs like Selacryn® will represent a significant advance over current diuretics.

4

Rheumatoid arthritis

THE TYPES OF ARTHRITIS I've gone over so far had special features, or characteristics, that made them easy to recognize. They usually appeared at a certain age, involved certain joints, and the attacks came on the same way in most people. Fairly standard treatments would work for everyone with that type of arthritis. Rheumatoid arthritis, or RA for short, isn't like that.

This form of arthritis really is different for virtually everyone who has it. It doesn't follow any single set pattern. The treatments are different, too, for each person. In the first part of this chapter, I'll go through the range of what RA can cause. Then I'll go into why all this happens, and what can be done about it. Throughout this chapter, there are a few things you should keep in mind at all times: (1) RA in any one person will be a combination of some of the things RA can cause; not every problem occurs in everyone. (2) RA can start at any age, from childhood to very old age, but it usually stops 10-20 years after it starts; any arthritis that's left is usually wear and tear arthritis on joints that had been damaged previously by RA. A disease doctors call "juvenile RA" probably is not the same as RA in a child, and isn't taken up in this book. (3) Any useful treatment for RA must work on the basic cause of the disease.

As you might expect from the name of the illness, the most common feature of RA is arthritis. Unlike the types of arthritis so far, joint stiffness is one of the main problems and often appears before any pain or swelling. Like wear arthritis, the stiffness is worse in the morning, and is better after mild use. Unlike wear arthritis, though, the stiffness is often severe. The lubricating fluid in the joints in RA is bad, and tends to cause both the joints to freeze up, and the easy wearing down on the teflon caps with time. Any joint that has two bones moving across each other can be involved in RA, but the wrists, bases of the fingers, knees, and hips are the most common areas. The arthritis usually appears on both sides at the same time, as well. The wrist is particularly susceptible because it doesn't have a joint the way the other bones in our body do. It's made from a string of bones, the way some belts and necklaces are made from a string of plates. This allows the wrist to bend in all directions, and fold over on itself. But it also means that there are many joints, all slipping over one another. A joint that slides like that relies heavily on its lubricant. When this is poor, as in RA, the teflon surfaces wear quickly.

Another reasonably typical thing about the arthritis in RA is a special type of joint swelling. In wear arthritis or gout, one or another joint may swell on occasion, but it's just that—swelling on occasion, with nothing in between. The bone around the joint may be enlarged from spur formation, but the joint bag itself usually isn't swollen. In RA, the problem is in the lining of the joint, and that lining is usually swollen. There may or may not be free fluid in the joint, but the lining often feels "thick." Joints with no lining, like those between most of the pelvic or spinal bones, can't develop RA, Some of the joints in the neck behind the bones and the joint between the base of the head and the neck do have a lining and can develop RA.

A few unusual joints can be involved that aren't affected in most other forms of arthritis. The first of these is the jaw. The joint between the jawbone and the head that lets you open and close your mouth can be affected on one or both sides. This makes it very painful to chew or talk. The joint can swell and feel like a swollen gland, even though it isn't. If only this joint is affected by arthritis, though, it doesn't mean the problem has to be RA. Another odd joint where RA shows up is in the voicebox. There are joints that let the internal parts move about, so we can speak and breathe. When the problem is mild, hoarseness is present. When it's more severe, it actually hurts to talk, with the pain very low in the throat. Your air goes through the voicebox as it goes in and out of the lungs, and there is no way around it. If arthritis of these joints is bad, the voicebox can freeze closed and keep you from breathing. When this joint is involved, special action may be needed to prevent this.

In addition to the lining of the joints thickening, the bag that surrounds the joint can weaken as well. The ballooning of these bags is what actually causes the joints to seem swollen. In the knee, the ballooning and weakening can be especially bad. The bag may enlarge out behind the knee and work its way down the leg. The large sac that results can break open easily, releasing its contents into the leg. Unlike the normal joint, the bag contains activated detergents and other destructive materials that are present in joints involved with RA. When it breaks open, sudden and severe pain results. This is called a popliteal cyst rupture, and is easy to confuse with a severe sprain or blood clot.

A number of other problems can appear in RA. They are not the result of the arthritis. Instead, both the arthritis and these other things are the result of the basic thing happening in RA. One of the commonest of these additional problems is the rheumatoid nodule. This is a lump, one-fourth to two inches in size, that may appear in many places in the body. It's most easily seen in the skin, where you can also feel it. It's firm, doesn't hurt, and may be a little red. It usually appears in areas of mild injury, and is therefore often found on the shins or just below the elbows. The nodule is the result of a damaged area in a small artery. When the artery is small, and the other arteries around it are OK, not much besides the nodule happens. Sometimes in RA, though, many arteries are badly damaged. This may develop to the point where not enough blood can get through to fill the needs of some parts of the body. When this happens, small, usually painful black spots appear on the fingers or toes. These are areas of skin that have lost so much blood that they have died. The same thing can happen in the brain, causing a stroke, or in the heart. Fortunately, problems this severe aren't common in RA.

Even when the blood supply remains adequate, the nodule can pose problems by the pressure it exerts. If the nodule forms in a nerve cable, the pressure alone can partially or completely stop the entire nerve from working. If the pressure is great enough, or if the nerve loses its blood supply, the nerve may die. More often an imbalance of nerve signals going to the brain results, and a constant painful feeling is present.

The nodules do not play a role in the arthritis itself. However, as the arthritis gets better or worse, so do the nodules, if the arthritis is due to RA, and not wear and tear.

A great many other problems can occur in RA, which I won't mention here in detail since they won't add to your understanding of what goes wrong and what to do about RA. For all these problems, including the ones that follow, remember that not everyone gets them. Each of these other problems can also occur without arthritis. By tradition, the disease is not called RA then, though it usually is the same disease, even without the arthritis! It's the same sheep in a different coat.

Occasionally, people who have RA have a fever and lymph node enlargement as well. This is usually present only when a large number of joints are involved though they don't need to be severely affected. This feature of RA is particularly common in children and in people over 60. If a sample is taken from one of the nodes, it may resemble some cancers, though it isn't.

The cables that hook the muscles up to the bones they move slide in liners or sheaths that are similar to the inside of a joint bag. In RA, the lining of these sheaths for the cables (tendons) is rough and doesn't produce a good lubricating fluid. As a result the tendons have the same stiffness problems that the joints do. They can fray and break.

The last feature of RA that's important is dry eyes. It's important because, when it's present, one of the newer treatments for RA usually won't work. The dry eyes problem is actually more than just that. The first thing to go wrong is excessive watering of the eyes. Later, the eyes don't produce tears. The reason for this sequence of events is that the eyes have two tear systems. The first one to go bad is always the one that produces a small, steady flow of tears. The second is there only to make a waterfall to wash out the eyes when there's too much for the first system to handle. If the first system stops working, the second one works all the time. When it's on, there's no way to set it for a small flow. Later this one fails, and the eyes make no tears at all. In addition, the saliva glands in the mouth often stop working, and the mouth becomes very dry as well. The medical term for this is Sjogren's syndrome. There's one last thing to be careful about. The usual cause of dry eyes (especially the first, heavy tearing state) is the birth control pill. When it's due to the pill, it doesn't have any effect on which treatments can be used.

The Characteristics of RA

There are several features that would make you think an arthritis problem might be RA: (1) Joint stiffness and swelling in several large joints, particularly at the bases of the fingers, toes, and wrists. (2) Pain and swelling along the tendons. (3) Firm lumps at the elbow, shin, and back of the hand. (4) Onset of the arthritis under 40 or over 65. (5) Dry eyes and mouth.

What causes all this mess? What's going wrong in RA that makes so many things go bad?

The story centers around how our body defends itself against infection. Infection itself usually isn't the direct cause of the RA. Instead the problem comes from something going wrong with the way our body defends itself against infections. Sometimes our defense system is overly activated and destroys much more than just the bugs causing the infection. Despite this overkill, the defenses aren't accurate enough to get rid of all the bugs. Then the infection lasts for years, as does the accidental destruction of parts of the body. Arthritis can develop either because the bugs are in the joint lining to begin with, or because material from the dead bugs settles there, bringing the body's destructive forces along with them.

Let's start at the beginning. There's a very basic idea behind infections. Many other forms of life can live inside our bodies. There are four types of these other forms of life. The first is bacteria. These very tiny animals that exist complete in one cell are an independent, self-contained life form. These animals live on our body's fluids. They cause things like strep throats, pneumonias, or skin infections. The second type, less often a problem for us, is a tiny plant, called a fungus. These also live on body fluids, usually in the skin. The third is worms. These are common throughout much of the world. They are fairly large, usually living in our intestines. Finally, there are the viruses. Viruses are chemicals, at least when they are outside our body. They're a very complex chemical with an outer coat, or envelope. Inside this is a long piece of code—like magnetic tape that goes into a tape recorder or computer. On the tape is a long line of instructions that goes into our body's own machinery. By supplying the coded tape, the viruses can literally take over individual cells in our body to make more of themselves. They make copies of the tape, more envelopes, put them together, and release them into our blood or the air. Sometimes the cells in the body where the viruses are made can recover from all this, sometimes not.

If we are to survive in this world, our body must have defenses against all of these other forms of life. If we didn't, any one of them could take over our body and kill us quickly. So obviously, we've got the defenses, and so do all other animals and plants. The simplest of these defenses is a special detergent. Bacteria and viruses are made with different materials in the walls of their cells or envelopes than our cells have. As a result, we make a group of special detergents that will dissolve the bacteria, and not ourselves. This system works pretty well. Some animals rely on this system alone. However, it isn't very refined. When you get to bodies as complex as a fish, bird, or human being, the detergent system has trouble telling what it should and shouldn't dissolve. A second system is added in to recognize what should and shouldn't be inside our bodies with pinpoint accuracy. Each cell, each unit in our body has a structure to it. The outside of every cell is just like a building: each brick or shingle is neatly in place. There are windows, wires going in, water lines, and all that. Incredible as this may sound, your body is able to recognize each feature separately, and know it should be there. In addition, your body can recognize things that shouldn't be there at all. How many of these things can it recognize? Literally billions. How does it do it? It uses chemicals. The chemicals are like an alarm attached to a hook. When the hook comes in contact with one thing and only one thing that the body doesn't normally have, it sticks in place. Once the hook is firmly in place, the alarm goes on. The alarm makes the detergent system activate, as well as other things that help destroy whatever the hook is attached to. Remember that for any one hook, there is only one thing it will attach to—for example a certain type of door knob. Any door with that knob will get hooked. Another door, otherwise identical, but with a different knob won't be touched. There are billions of these hook and alarm combinations in our body. If something comes in from the outside and your body doesn't have a hook that will stick to it, then nothing happens, until either your body comes up with a new hook, or until the detergent system destroys it using its general abilities along that line. When the hook and alarm system does attach to something, the body recognizes it as foreign and tries to destroy it. This will happen even if the hook attaches to something that should be within the body. Once the alarm is turned on, whatever it is attached to is labeled "foreign" and marked for destruction.

Can we make any type of hook at all? No, we can't. The hooks we make are determined by heredity. The plans and blueprints for the hooks are there before we're born. All our body can do is call up the plans from storage. They can be changed a little, but not much. If the basic plans aren't there then we can't make a hook and alarm assem-

HOOK AND ALARM ASSEMBLIES AT WORK

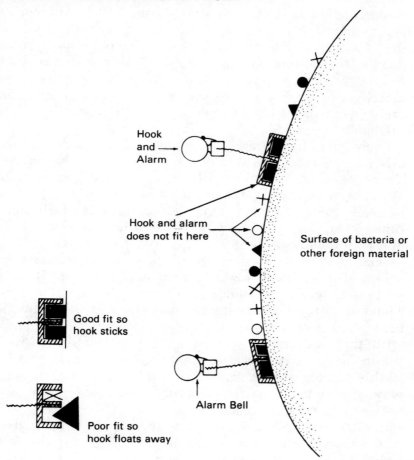

bly to attach. Usually, a large number of hooks won't be made unless something is around for them to be made against. There's another restriction on which hook and alarm assemblies can be made. One thing we don't want to happen is for the hooks to be able to attach to things that should be in our own body. It sounds simple: just be sure we don't inherit blueprints for hooks that can attach to our bodies. It isn't so simple. Remember that blueprints can change a little, and mistakes are then made. Over the last 100,000 years, the viruses and bacteria have gotten good at resembling our own bodies. This makes it tough to recognize them as foreign and still keep the hooks from attaching to us. For you to see how these unwanted hooks are prevented, I'll have to explain a little more about how the hooks are made.

Each type of hook and alarm assembly is made within a cell in the body, usually one type of assembly per cell. These cells are either white blood cells called *lymphocytes*, or similar cells. When the assemblies of one particular cell are in demand, this cell duplicates itself many times over, so that many new factories are made. This gives the body a large supply of the particular hook assembly it needs. The white blood cell that makes these assemblies carries a few on its surface. These are its label so that other white blood cells can tell what it's doing. That's how the body keeps things in line. Still other white blood cells, called suppressor cells, compare the hooks with their catalog of what the body normally has in it. White blood cells that start making hooks against things in this catalog are destroyed, or at least kept in line. That way, the body keeps from having any sizable number of hooks directed against itself.

In RA, several things go wrong with this system. Alarms are turned on in the blood vessels of the joint lining, causing damage to this lining and the production of a poor lubricating fluid. Hooks are also made against the body's own normal materials, and the suppressor cells are unable to control this. This also occurs primarily in the joint lining, creating further damage to the lubrication system, and rapid joint wear. These activated alarms also cause the blood vessels that line the joint bag to grow in size and branch out. A P-G type of chemical seems to do part of this, but other chemicals are also involved. The new blood vessels form throughout the bag, but the largest arteries are at the base, near the bone. These are the areas where the most P-G is produced, and where the most new blood vessels form. These new vessels apply pressure on and under the teflon cap. In addition, the P-G produced in the new blood vessels flows into the bone around them, and causes the bone to lose its marble. As a result, these vessels appear to eat into the joint. Actually they chemically dissolve it. Once this bone is damaged, the teflon cap can't be produced properly, and the damage from poor lubrication can't be repaired completely.

Why should these hooks be made in the joints and not throughout the entire body? Sometimes they are present throughout the whole body, and RA frequently is a disease that affects the entire body at once. At other times, though, the hook and alarm assemblies really are just in the joints. There are only two reasons the hooks are made. The first is that a white blood cell senses something

BLOOD VESSELS "EAT" INTO BONE

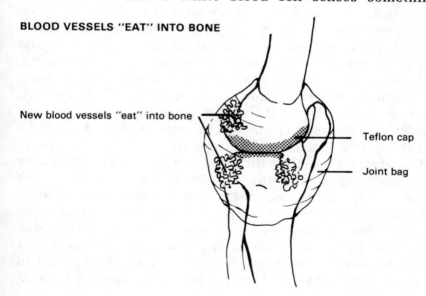

New blood vessels "eat" into bone

Teflon cap

Joint bag

nearby that its hook will catch on. The second is that the suppressor white blood cell is not able to stop the production of assemblies that should not be made. Both possibilities bear directly on RA.

Either way, the alarm assemblies cause damage to the joints and other parts of the body by settling out in the walls of the blood vessels. The joints are the most susceptible to this because of the arrangement of blood vessels in the wall of the joint bag. It acts like a filter that traps the alarms. Once they are on, they activate the detergent system, which causes both pain and swelling. In the joint bag, it also makes quite a change in the type of lubricant the bag produces. The properties of the lubricant that make it work well under pressure disappear. Any other place that the activated alarms settle out are also damaged by the detergent. They, however, tend to hurt less, and are noticed less.

Back to the possible causes of RA that I just mentioned, the first of these really comes down to the presence of an infection. If the infection were limited to the joints, then the hooks and alarms would be primarily produced there. If not, then they would be produced throughout the body. The general possibility of an infection as a cause of RA has received a great deal of attention over the past years. To date, no one has found the infection(s) that cause RA. But we do know that if there is one there, it won't be easy to find. One reason is that the infection doesn't have to be in the joints. It can be elsewhere in the body. Then parts of the bugs, even after they die, and the hooks and alarms the body makes to tag the bugs for destruction can combine and settle out in the joints, among other places. Once this happens, the body mounts an attack against the bugs—dead or alive—in the joints. For the attack, the body uses two main things. The first is the detergent that tries to dissolve the bugs. The second, which is called in by the detergent as it activates, is a type of garbage truck—a special type of white blood cell (the one involved in gout attacks) that scoops up the tagged bug and digests or kills it. Both of these means of attack aren't too accurate and anything nearby, including your own body, can be hurt as well. This usually helps heal or control the infection. If the bugs or parts of them after they die are carried away from the main site of infection and settle in the joints, then the body's attack destroys or damages the joints without really helping fight the infection. Sometimes the infection really is in the joints, among other places, and the body is actively attacking an infection there. This type of thing sometimes leads to a disease that can look just like RA. Then, the body can't tag the bugs accurately so it can't make quite the right hooks. It even seems to make a mistake and produce hooks that tag the blood vessels in the joint bag, instead of the bugs at all! As a result, the infection doesn't clear up, and the joints are hurt.

How many times is RA due to an infection? We just don't know. Part of the reason is that, when we realize our mistake in calling a certain type of infection RA, from then on, we separate that type of arthritis out from RA itself. These diseases, like *Reiter's* disease, (RA with peeling skin and pain on urinating) and *Whipple's* disease (RA with intestinal problems) are now called infections, rather than a form of RA. How many people are now said to have RA when they actually have a treatable infection as the cause of their arthritis? I can only guess that the number is high. The arthritis from this sort of infection (when it can be proven to be an infection) looks just like "typical RA." How to tell them apart is a difficult task, and one you'll have to trust to your physician. If you have this type of arthritis, 6-12 months of antibiotics is often required. The fact that you have this type of infection in the first place means that your body is having trouble making effective hooks. It'll need lots of help over a long period of time to be cured. You may also need to use the drugs mentioned later in this chapter that stimulate white blood cells to do a better job.

The second possible cause of RA is a problem with the *suppressor cells*. These cells are needed—and we have them normally—to stop any white blood cells from going too far if they start making hooks that will attach to the body's normal parts. This second cause is very closely tied in with the first one I told you about resulting from chronic infection. Because of the similarities between the bugs causing infections and ourselves, hooks that attach to our normal structures tend to be produced during many infections. In addition, the longer an infection has been present, more refined and accurate hooks are made against the old bugs that cause it. As better hooks are made, production of the old ones is shut down. The suppressor cells probably play a part in this, too. A defect in suppressor cell function both leaves us open for attack by our own defenses and removes the fine tuning from the defenses as well, making them less effective.

How does the suppressor cell do this? The suppressor cell makes hooks of its own, similar to the other white blood cells. The ones that the suppressor cells make will attach to other hooks, made by the other white blood cells *if* these others will attach to the body's own structures, or if their production should be shut down, in favor of a later model. The white blood cells that make hooks also have them attached to their surface. The suppressor cell's hooks attach to these while they are on the surface of the white blood cell making them. This lets the suppressor cell find the other white blood cells that aren't working quite right. It either destroys them, or at least, stops them from making more of themselves and more hooks to react with your own body. The suppressor cells also release something similar to a hook and alarm assembly into the blood that works on white blood cells at some distance from the release point, to accomplish the same thing.

There's another wrinkle in the works, though. White blood cells will keep making hook and alarm assemblies as long as there are things around that the hooks can attach to. The hooks on the surface of the white blood cells also latch on to parts of the bugs that cause the

SUPPRESSOR CELL OPERATION

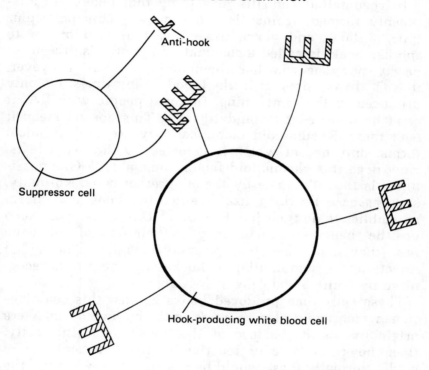

Anti-hook

Suppressor cell

Hook-producing white blood cell

infection. This triggers the cell to make more hook and alarm assemblies. As long as there is something— anything—around that will match the hook that the white blood cell is currently making, more assemblies are cranked out. If, by mistake, the hooks are made that can also attach to a natural part of the body, there is always something around to stimulate the cell to make hooks. If the suppressor cells are not working, this mistake continues for a very long time. This also means RA can start as an infection either in the joints or elsewhere in the body, and then last long after the infection is gone if hooks originally designed to combat the infection attach to other things in the body as well.

In rheumatoid arthritis, one thing that hooks are mistakenly formed against is other hooks. This particular type of hook and alarm assembly, that will attach to another hook, is called a rheumatoid factor. It's present in nearly everyone who has rheumatoid arthritis. However, it isn't always present in the blood. Many times, it's only produced in the joint lining. In some people with RA, it can't be detected by standard tests. This doesn't mean it isn't there. Rheumatoid factor can have several chemical forms, only one of which is detected by the usual tests. How does this rheumatoid factor come about? One possibility is that it's made by the suppressor cells. Normally, suppressor cells don't use free-floating hook and alarm assemblies to do their job. However, if they just can't keep up, the rheumatoid factor may be their way of doing the best they can. The other possibility is that, during an infection, the combination of hooks with bugs was recognized by white blood cells as foreign.

These cells then produced hooks against this combination, which could also combine with the hooks that were originally on the surface of the bugs, alone. Indirectly, then, hooks capable of reacting with other hooks were made. Normally these would be destroyed. However, if the suppressor cells weren't up to their job, these new, rheumatoid factor hooks would continue to be made, even after the infection is gone. In this situation, the rheumatoid factor would actually interfere with the body's defenses against infection. Restoring the ability of the suppressor cells to stop the production of rheumatoid factor would help both the infection and the arthritis at once.

Does the rheumatoid factor mean that RA isn't really due to an infection, but is due to this factor instead? Quite the opposite. Rheumatoid factor appears in many chronic infections of known cause, even if no arthritis is present.

Treatments for RA

The problems that people have from RA cover such a wide range that the treatment has to be done on a very individual basis. The difficulties that the treatments themselves can cause can also be significant. The risks and discomforts resulting from the treatments must be considered in proper balance with the problems that RA can cause. It won't help in the long run if you use treatments sparingly, then wind up crippled for the rest of your life. Nor does it make sense to use a treatment that can cause cancer if your arthritis is mild and your joints aren't being destroyed.

All the successful treatments for RA are directed at the basic things that go wrong in this disease. Most of them work on the things that cause poor lubrication of the joint, and the destruction of the bone under the joint by growing blood vessels. A few of the treatments—those that work on the suppressor cells—may actually work on the basic cause of RA. At this time, there is no treatment that tries to clear up any underlying infection that may have been the cause of the RA initially. For many people with RA, no one treatment is a perfect answer, and many times several are used in combination.

Because of the problem with joint lubrication and excessive wear on the teflon cap, one basic factor in all treatments of RA is moderate joint exercise without undue overuse. The basic exercises are listed in the chapter on wear arthritis. The important things to remember are: (1) frequent, mild joint exercise helps preserve the joint and keep it lubricated; no use at all will freeze it; (2) actions that cause quick, sudden strains on a joint involved with RA must be avoided. If the hands are involved, sewing, piano or other musical instrument playing, baseball, tennis and carpentry usually should be avoided. If the knees or ankles are involved, running, walking on rough ground, kneeling, or jumping have to go. You can't cause a joint affected with RA to improve by "working it hard." You'll only destroy it.

One of the older treatments for RA, which I do not recommend, carries the "don't use the joint" idea to the extreme. The treatment is simply complete rest in bed until the RA is over (usually 8-15 years). This supposedly protects the joints against damage until the RA is gone. There are a few problems with it, though. It's a hard way to live one's life but more than that the bones lose their marble rapidly, and the electrical forces under the joints decrease. As a result, a poor teflon cap is formed. Also, destruction of the joints isn't only due to movement and wear. New blood vessels cut into the bone under the teflon cap, independent of movement, and also destroy the joint. The lack of movement lets the joints freeze. Rest is good for RA, but don't get carried away with the idea.

There are no vitamins or special diet for RA, or any sort of arthritis. You do need an adequate vitamin and protein intake, but an excess won't help. If you don't think you get enough vitamins, use the One A Day® or similar daily multivitamins (not the high potency) and take one a day. Don't use the protein supplements that are on the market at health food stores. These supplements do not add useful protein to your diet or body. Your body cannot use protein they contain as a replacement for proper dietary protein. If you do have a problem along these lines, there are special protein supplements for this purpose: Casec® and Citrotein® are two good ones.

Most people with RA begin treatment with a drug that cuts down on P-G production in the lining of the joints and tendons. This reduces the pain and stiffness considerably. Over the long term, however, it also decreases the formation of new blood vessels that eat into the bones near the joints. To a lesser extent, they also cut down on the ability of the white blood cells to make hook and alarm assemblies. Not all the drugs that do this are free of trouble or safe for long-term use. In general, Clinoril® 150-400 mg twice daily, offers the best compromise. If you can't use this for some reason, alternatives are discussed in the last chapter. If you have a mild case of RA, Clinoril® may be the only drug you need to feel perfectly normal. In judging what's normal, remember the final thing to judge is joint stiffness, not pain. The best time to judge this is first thing in the morning. Also, remember to wait two weeks before gauging the full effect of Clinoril®, which should be taken daily, whether your joints ache or not.

Most people with RA should take a second medicine along with Clinoril® in order to reduce pain and stiffness and prevent destruction of the joints. Since P-G's play an important role in the joint damage, controlling their production with Clinoril® will help prevent the progression of the arthritis. The P-G's, however, aren't the only chemical released when alarms target something for destruction. The alarms also attract white blood cells to digest and dissolve the thing that's tagged as well as activate a detergent system near the thing tagged. Several other drugs seem to affect these things as well as cut down on the production of the hook and alarm assemblies. These drugs, like Clinoril®, are taken on a continuous basis. They take longer to work, and have some greater potential difficulties than Clinoril®.

For everyone with RA, except the person who is only mildly affected, the first choice among these additional drugs is Plaquanil®. In addition to working in the ways mentioned in the preceeding paragraph, this drug is an antibiotic. Whether it works in this capacity against RA isn't known. Usually Plaquanil® can't be used alone for RA because it isn't very effective in relieving pain. For people who can't use Clinoril® and its related drugs at all, Plaquanil® becomes the first choice. This drugs requires quite a long time to work its full effect, so be sure to try it for at least two months before deciding whether to continue using it or not. I recommend this drug because of its relative freedom from undesirable effects. In very large amounts and in people who, for hereditary reasons, retain it in the body more than usual, it can cause problems with eyesight. Color vision and the ability to see fine details may be worsened or lost. If the drug is stopped for a while, everything returns to normal, and it can be restarted. Most of the people who have had this side effect have taken 500 mg or more a day while the amount recommended for treatment in RA is 250 mg daily for 5 days a week. This dosage avoids the eye problem completely. Occasionally 1 tablet 7 days a week is needed. If children with RA use this drug, they need much lower dosage because of possible heart problems. Anyone with significant psoriasis probably shouldn't use this drug since it may make the psoriasis much worse. A related drug, Aralen®, has also been used and is also approved by the FDA for use against RA. Although Aralen® is probably a little more effective than Plaquanil®, the undesirable side effects are much worse and, in general, this drug should not be used in place of Plaquanil®. Plaquanil® remains in the body for many months or years after you stop using it, and therefore will continue to help your RA long after you've stopped using it. Since Plaquanil® takes so long to start working, due to the build-up required, sometimes it helps to use 500 mg of it a day for the first month only.

In doing its job for RA, Plaquanil® works on the white blood cells as they try to make hook and alarm assemblies and try to respond to the activated alarms. The other drugs now available for use as a "next step" after Clinoril® don't do this. These drugs partially take apart the hook and alarm assemblies, and partially stop some of the chemicals the white blood cells, primarily the scavenger type, release from working. They do only a partial job of this, so they aren't very effective. But they do help and their benefits are in addition to what you get from either Clinoril® or Plaquanil®. They can also be used along with either of these drugs. These drugs are gold-containing chemicals that can only be taken by injection. Usually 50 mg is used once a week, with an extra amount during the first week of use or so. Unfortunately, all of the half-dozen gold injection drugs have the same, fairly frequent undesirable effects. All can cause real problems with skin rash, anemia (low blood count), kidney damage, and allergic reactions as well as a whole host of rare reactions. Unfortunately, these gold drugs remain in the body for a long time after the injections are stopped, and long after they have ceased to help the RA. As a result, if a reaction occurs, it tends to last a very long time. Finally, another useful drug for RA, *penacillamine*, should not be used, if at all possible, for several months to a year after gold injections. All of the following gold injections are equally good, require 2-4 months to work and have the same problems: Solgonal® (gold thioglucose); Auralin®, Auropin®, Aurosan® (gold thiosulfate); Aurothiomalate®; Aurothioblycanide®.

For people with RA who have had inadequate relief with Clinoril® and Plaquanil®, gold injections can provide reasonable additional help with a moderate risk of ill effects. Within the next few years, however, another "gold-based" drug will be appearing, which is completely different from the injections currently available. This drug is *auranofin* (a trademark isn't assigned yet), and is taken two or three times a day as a tablet. It generally works within a month to 6 weeks, and provides a great deal of help for this type of arthritis. Unlike the injections, *auranofin* works on the white blood cells and prevents their activation by the alarms, prevents their production of hooks, and prevents their release of chemicals that damage the joints. When this drug becomes available, it will probably replace Plaquanil® as the drug to use along with Clinoril®, as well as making the injectable gold drugs completely undesirable. Because *auranofin* is completely different chemically from the injections, there have not been the same problems with serious bad effects. In addition, it can probably be used with or before *penacillamine*. Because *auranofin* is similar to Plaquanil® in a number of its actions, using the two in combination is likely to give less help than other combinations with Plaquanil®.

What do you do if the drugs already mentioned don't work well enough? *First, remember that any medicine or treatment for RA cannot reverse actual damage to the joint.* If that is your problem—and you may need the help of your doctor to decide that—no treatment, except possibly joint replacement or fusion will help you. However, if the problem is that the RA is still progressing (and that's often the case) there are several other treatments to be used. These are all somewhat more effective than the treatments I've outlined so far, but they have greater difficulties as well. From here on, I'll go over them in their order of both increasing effectiveness and, unfortunately, increasing danger and difficulty. None of these treatments, with one exception, does anything for the underlying disease. Some of them may actually worsen it.

The first of these is *penacillamine* (Cupramine®). This treatment, recently approved by the FDA for use in RA, can be used along with Clinoril® and Plaquanil® but should not be used with any of the gold-containing drugs (except *auranofin* perhaps), since it inactivates them, and increases their undesirable effects. It can be used follow-ing the use of the gold drugs, but if at all possible, a several month gap should be allowed. You are much more likely to have problems from *penacillamine* if it's used after gold, because the gold remains in the body. The longer you wait, the better. *Penacillamine* can be used with any of the following treatments though. The drug works in several ways. It takes apart the hook and alarm assembly, so the alarm can't be triggered anymore. It may stop the entry of white blood cells into the joint, cut down on P-G production, and inactivate the chemicals the blood vessels make to dissolve the bone and teflon cap as they try to "grow" into it. As you would guess from what it does, *penacillamine* is fairly effective for RA since it hits several things that go wrong at once. Its bad effects limit its use. There are several common and important ones, and literally a hundred or more rare ones. The common problems are skin rash and kidney damage. In general, the more of the drug that's used, the greater the chance of problems, and the worse they are. To keep the amount low, use it along with other drugs, like Clinoril® and Plaquanil®. In part, the kidney problems are the result of the disassembly of the hooks and alarms. The disas-sembled parts come out in the urine, and can damage the kidney if their concentration is high. So drinking lots of fluids (or using water pills—diuretics) will help prevent the kidney problems. *Penacillamine* will tend to deplete the body of iron, copper, and trace metals. Do not take supplements of these while using *penacillamine*, and be sure your vitamins don't include minerals. These supple-ments increase the kidney damage quite a bit. If you need the supplements, stop taking the *penacillamine* at that time. If a skin rash develops, remember that it may have been due to the prior use of gold. If so, you may be able to use *penacillamine* 6-12 months later without a problem.

The usual dosage of *penacillamine* is 1 to 4 capsules a

day. Start low if possible, and wait 10 days to 2 weeks before each increase. *Penacillamine* works quickly compared to gold-containing drugs and Plaquanil®, but it still requires time to work. The relatively fast action, though, means that you can use it briefly while starting Plaquanil® and waiting for it to work.

Next in the scale of effectiveness and risk is the one treatment that may actually help cure people of the basic problem behind RA. If the difficulties with it can be removed, this treatment may become the first choice for RA. Most of the drugs mentioned work on the white blood cells to one extent or another. All of them, except possibly Plaquanil®, depress the normal functions of the white blood cell. A new group of drugs stimulates the white blood cells, and these are proving to be quite effective in the treatment of RA. If the white blood cells are the seat of the problem in RA, why stimulate them? Remember that not all white blood cells are the same. Some make the hook and alarm assemblies. Others control the cells that make them and can prevent the hooks from being made. These new drugs don't stimulate the cells that make the hooks and alarms, but do stimulate the suppressor cells that can correct the situation when the wrong ones are made. There is yet another type of white blood cell in our body: It helps identify infections and tell other white blood cells what type of hook to make. This cell is also stimulated by these drugs. This way, they actually aid the body in fighting any infection that might be there.

Levamisole is the drug that has had the most testing in RA to date. Trials have shown that this drug works quite well in RA, and is able to decrease joint swelling and pain a great deal. It may also be able to prevent involvement of new joints as well, but it hasn't been used long enough to be sure. In overall effectiveness, this drug appears to be a little more effective than *penacillamine*. It can be used in combination with any of the drugs for RA. However, gold drugs (except *auranofin*) and to a lesser extent, *penacillamine* have similar undersirable effects. If problems occur when *levamisole* is used with these, it may be difficult to determine which is causing the problem. With *levamisole*, about 5% of people with RA who took it daily had severe anemia. The anemia appears to be related to how much of the drug is taken, though, and it looks like it will be possible to use it only a few days a week to avoid this problem but still control the arthritis. A second problem was that everyone with dry eyes (Sjogren's syndrome) who used *levamisole* developed a severe skin rash, and had to stop taking the drug. These people had used the drug daily, and we still don't know what would happen if they used less of the drug.

It looks as if the proper dosage of *levamisole* is from 100 mg once a week to 150 mg three times a week. Even at lower dosages—25-50 mg once a week—some benefit is there. Some very special cautions, too complex to go into here, must be taken when the drug is used in children or people with "juvenile rheumatoid arthritis." The drug, marketed as Ripercol® (American Cyanamid), is not approved for human use by the FDA as yet. Approval to date has only been for sheep. Although the drug is marketed as an antibiotic against worms, there isn't anything to suggest that it works this way in RA.

The second drug in this group, which is approved by the FDA for human use but not specifically for RA, is Tagamet®. Although originally marketed for ulcers and related intestinal problems, this drug has shown a number of similarities to *levamisole* with regard to white blood cells. There has been less experience with it than with *levamisole* and it appears to be less effective, but probably is in the same "range" as Plaquanil®. Unlike the other drugs, it is remarkably safe to use and can be used along with all the other drugs for RA. Dosage is 2-4 tablets a day.

At this point, we really don't know where *levamisole* and Tagamet® fit in the picture of treatments for RA. The basic fact that they seem to work right at the cause for RA makes them extremely desirable drugs to use. Even with its current problems, *levamisole* in adults may come as a close second to Plaquanil® and *auranofin* as a recommended treatment for RA. If Tagamet® proves more effective than it seems at present, its safety would make it an alternative to Clinoril® or Plaquanil® as well. Preliminary results don't indicate it is effective enough for that.

All the treatments I've gone over so far have their good and bad sides. The problems with them are something of a chance happening: not everyone gets the problem and some people have no trouble at all. With the last two groups of drugs to follow, this is not the case. Everyone who uses them has serious problems or runs serious risks. The severity of the problem differs from person to person and, to a large extent, depends on dosage and duration of use.

The first of these treatments involves cortisone-like drugs. The natural forms, *cortisone* and *hydrocortisone*, are never used due to severe salt and water retention that occurs. To avoid this, synthetic forms are used. All the synthetic forms still share all the other undesirable effects of cortisone. For a given amount of cortisone-like benefits, you always get a proportional amount of cortisone-like ill effects. For reasons of cost, *prednisone* is the drug usually used.

What does *prednisone* do? It tells your body to make a natural material that works like Clinoril® and aspirin, but is much more effective. So indirectly, *prednisone* decreases P-G production throughout the body. This decreases the joint pain, swelling, stiffness, and growth of new blood vessels into the bone under the joint. Unfortunately, the natural material is so much better at this than Clinoril® that it also stops new bone formation and repair, skin repair, and white blood cell activity. These last actions lead to a great number of ill effects in everyone who uses *prednisone*. The more you use, the worse they are.

Since much of what *prednisone* does can be accomplished by the other drugs, the use of *prednisone* is quite limited in RA. Its use primarily centers around its ability to depress the action of the white blood cells (both the scavenger type and those involved with the hooks). Most of the other drugs don't do too much of this. *Prednisone* is used when RA involves the eye, arteries, brain, and nerves. These are all very serious problems, and here the benefits of *prednisone* usually outweigh the risks. *Prednisone* can be used for severe arthritis where joint destruction is progressing rapidly, as well. It works quickly, and is particularly good as a temporary measure until the other drugs, which take longer to act, start in. Very rarely, it has to be continued long term.

Some physicians use a tiny amount of *prednisone*—2.5-5 mg daily—for RA. This is a mistake. The body naturally produces the equal of 7.5 mg of *prednisone* a day, almost all of it in the morning. If you take small amounts during the day, your body simply makes that much less. You haven't added anything to what's already there and this causes a problem! Over a period of years, particularly if the *prednisone* is taken after noon, your body will stop making its own cortisone, and may lose the ability to make more. So if you get into a situation where your body requires more cortisone, your body will no longer be able to make it naturally.

What about joint injections of *prednisone*? Unlike the situation with wear arthritis, a substantial amount of the cortisone injected does end up in the blood, because of the large number of irritated blood vessels in the joint lining. The injection does help the pain and swelling temporarily but also destroys the teflon cap and bone underneath. Joint injections may be of use after a bump or other injury to a joint involved by RA, but should not be used most of the time. In general, it should be limited to one injection a year. There's a complete discussion of *prednisone* and similar drugs in the last chapter that you may want to read.

The last group of drugs also acts on the white blood cell. They stop the production of hooks and alarms by most of the white blood cells that are actively making them. They also stop the action of the white blood cells that have hooks fixed to their surface, and use these as a "homing device" to find things. Some of these drugs will also prevent the body from "learning" to make new hooks to new bugs and other things that come along. This type of drug works both on the white blood cells that are "producing" the RA, and on the body's normal defenses as well. They are very effective in stopping the production of new blood vessels in the joints, preventing new joints from being involved, and decreasing swelling and stiffness. They also are good at preventing damage to the eyes, arteries, the brain, and nerves.

These drugs are quite effective, but at a very high price. They all significantly decrease the body's resistance against infection and some types of cancer. In general, the late development of cancer hasn't been a great problem with these drugs, but it has happened. Infection is a fairly common problem with them. The use of a drug like this in RA, where infection may be the underlying cause, isn't something that's done lightly. Most of them lower the white blood count, and some can cause a severe anemia. Some cause liver problems, and another (Cytoxan®) can cause severe bladder irritation.

Obviously, these drugs have great potential for help and harm. For a person who is losing his arteries, nerves, or brain from RA, these drugs can be very important. For people with severe and progressive RA, they may be needed to prevent total joint destruction, particularly if the joint at the base of the head is involved severely. Usually, when they are used, *prednisone* is used as well since the combination of the two reduces the dosage of each one that's required, and helps cut down on the unwanted effects. The dosages of these drugs, and *prednisone*, is always adjusted individually. With this last group of drugs, Cytoxan® is currently the most effective. Often, it can be used once a week to decrease the unwanted effects, along with lots of fluids to avoid bladder irritation. Usually these drugs are quite undesirable in children. In any event, they are a last resort but sometimes, it's a choice that must be made, and this must be decided individually.

Prednisone and related drugs are approved by the FDA for RA. Cytoxan® and the other similar drugs are approved by the FDA for other uses, not including RA.

There are two other forms of treatment for RA I would like to mention. The first focuses on the growth of new blood vessels that takes place in the joints and tendon sheaths that are involved with RA. The idea is to remove these chunks of blood vessels before they eat too deeply into the teflon cap and bone, or into the tendons. By and large, this form of treatment is undesirable, since opening the joint and cutting into the lining isn't the best treatment for an already damaged joint. After the operation, the joint is quite stiff and swollen, and may never regain full use. In addition, remember that in RA, the basic process is the formation of new blood vessels and swelling of the lining because of the action of white blood cells and the alarm assemblies they give off. Removing existing blood vessels won't change this, and it won't take too long for the lining to grow back to where it was before. By causing P-G's to be released, the operation actually stimulates this. Removing the lining creates two other problems. The lining is the source of the joint lubricant and the scavenger that picks up the chips of teflon that flake off. When the lining is removed, these are lost. There are exceptional circumstances where removing the lining is of use, but they're exceptional.

The final means of treatment is joint replacement. Sometimes in RA a joint is completely destroyed, either by RA itself, or by the wear arthritis that follows. For people with RA, the fingers, toes, knees, elbows, and hips are the main places where this occurs and something can be done. Except for the hip, replacement with an artificial joint is done only when nearly complete loss of use occurs. Hip replacements are much more successful, and can be done either for substantial loss of use, or severe pain. The hip, knee, and finger replacements are fairly well perfected now, and last around 10 years. The elbow joints are more experimental at this time, and only a few places attempt these replacements. A few centers have also been experimenting with ankle replacements as well, but the standard treatment for the ankle has been to fuse it together so it remains in a fixed position without too much pain. However, in RA, the ankle often does this on its own, and often this operation isn't needed.

The details on the joint replacements and coming developments in treatment are covered in the last chapter.

Take a look at the next chapter on diseases that look like RA. There are a substantial number that look very much like RA, but have much different causes and treatments. Since the treatments differ, and you're dealing with an illness that you'll have for some years to come, this chapter would be worth looking at.

When a good physician, using all available tests and opinions, makes a diagnosis of RA, he's doing well if he's right 75% of the time. Part of it is because so many diseases involve the same basic process as RA, and look the same for quite some time. Part of it is simply that we know more as time goes on and our tests get better. So, even if your diagnosis is definitely RA at this time, keep the look-alikes in mind.

5

Other inflammatory illnesses

IN THE PREVIOUS CHAPTERS ON GOUT AND RA, I talked about several ways the body seeks out and destroys things it doesn't want. The fact that our bodies can do this is what keeps us alive. These defenses are also the things that cause the problems of gout and RA. At this point, I'd like to go into these defenses a bit more, since they seem to be the direct cause of a number of other types of arthritis. The types of arthritis in this chapter are quite common, but they aren't talked about very often. Many people don't even know they exist. Unlike gout and wear arthritis, they often occur in young people.

In gout and wear arthritis, sudden joint pain and swelling occurs when crystals trigger the action of scavenger white blood cells. These scavenger cells are present throughout our body, and will eat up most anything that is "foreign." These scavengers don't need any hook and alarm assemblies, discussed in the chapter on RA, to trigger their action. (But if the hooks have attached to something, they do scavenge it better.) The cells recognize the basic structure of things they come in contact with. If the structure looks different from our own body, they literally swallow up the thing, or at least try to. Once the foreign particle is inside them, they chemically digest it away as best they can. How do these cells know where to go? They don't. They just wander aimlessly in the body. Well, almost. A large number of these cells are usually present in the blood, and in areas where blood is stored: the spleen and the bone marrow. When the body is under stress from infections, cortisone and other chemicals are released. These cause some white blood cells to leave the storage sites. Once in the blood, they remain there until they are allowed to leave by an area of infection or irritation. That way, scavenger cells are brought near the site of the problem. There they "home in" on the target. Normally these cells are moving around in every direction. If one of them hits something foreign, it releases a chemical that stops any other scavenger cell from moving away once it comes near. The hook and alarm assemblies can also do the same thing. At the same time that the alarms activate a detergent to dissolve out the unwanted stuff, they cause the detergent to make a chemical that also stops the scavenger cells in place. That way, the clean-up brigade is on hand to pick up what the detergents leave behind. The scavenger cells, though, cannot make hooks and alarms.

In rheumatoid arthritis and most of the other forms of arthritis in this chapter, the hook and alarm assemblies play the primary role. After tagging a substance or bug in the body for destruction, they can do several things, all at once. One of these is to help scavenger cells make their pick-up. The second is to activate a detergent system. The chemicals that make up the detergent system are present in the blood and other fluids of the body at all times. They are, however, "inactive." Unless an alarm that has been triggered by the attachment of its hook is nearby, these chemicals won't combine to form an active detergent. In addition, the detergent only works, or is active, near the site of the alarm. As it strays or is washed away, other chemicals in the blood destroy the detergent. This detergent plays an even more important role than it seems to play. The alarms use some of the chemicals in this detergent to attract the scavenger white blood cells, too. The detergent can also be activated in the absence of hooks and alarms. Some chemicals, particularly the ones bacteria have in their bodies, can directly activate the detergent in the vicinity of the bugs even without any hooks having been made against them.

The hooks serve one more purpose. The hooks, without the complete alarm assemblies attached, are present on still another type of white blood cell. They help this type of cell attach to foreign stuff and destroy it. This is a much more accurate type of hit than the scavenger cells make. This type of system is obviously very accurate and selective in what it destroys compared to the scavenger cells. The detergent system, as it's being activated, also attracts some of these hook-guided white blood cells to the area where they are needed as well.

It's a very complicated system. The central figure in all this is actually the detergent, since this is what is able to attract the two types of white blood cells in the first place, as well as the thing that does much of the actual destruction. None of this causes the pain or other sensations we feel with infections and injuries. That's caused by other chemicals, whose presence is usually either the result of the detergent system or of the scavenger white blood cells. Both of these activate other chemicals in the blood that cause the platelets or stop-leak particles (discussed in Chapter 3) to form clumps in the area of the stuff being destroyed. These trigger blood clots to form around the area, and release P-G's that open up little blood vessels in the surrounding area, and cause redness (from the color of the blood), warmth (from the heat of the blood and cells near the detergent), and pain (from the P-G's and other chemicals released). These last three things add up to *inflammation.* Inflammation is the end result of a long series of the body's reactions against something it considers foreign. It isn't the cause of anything. *Diseases where a great deal of inflammation is present throughout the body are called inflammatory diseases.* They include RA, and the types of arthritis to follow, as well as the diseases that can look like arthritis but really aren't.

Many of the inflammatory diseases are due to infections. Occasionally this infection is in the joints. More often, the infection is elsewhere in the body, and either the bugs or their destructive products combined with the hook and alarm assemblies settle out in the joints among other places and cause problems. The problems come from the white blood cells they attract and the detergent they activate.

Many virus infections in our bodies involve the joints with a mild inflammatory arthritis. Usually this isn't bad enough so that the joints actually swell. It does make them stiff in the mornings and increasingly painful throughout the day. The joints we use the most—the hands, fingers, wrists, and knees—are usually the most affected. This type of arthritis often appears just after the sniffles, sore throat, cough, and fever start. It's probably due to an actual infection of the joints—along with many other parts of the body—by the virus. As the virus releases its copies from the cells, they are broken down and cleaned up by the scavenger cells. This, plus the attachment of the hooks and alarms to the released viruses, causes the actual inflammation. In these early days of the illness, the hooks and alarms usually play a very minor role.

Sometimes the joint disease happens later on, after 10 days or more of being sick. Then, something else is going on. This type of virus arthritis is very common with the viruses that remain in the body for a long time. Most viruses don't hang around more than 10 days and are cleaned up and out of circulation after a week. However, several of them hang on better than that. In particular, the viruses that cause hepatitis (liver viruses), mononucleosis and related diseases, and herpes do this. They usually establish themselves in a few isolated places in the body. The hepatitis virus affects the liver. The mono virus and its relatives affect the liver, spleen, and lymph glands. Herpes usually affects the skin or nerves. From there, they can seed the blood both with complete viruses and with some of the parts from which the virus is made. With the hepatitis virus, often just the code tape, or the envelope, is given off alone. These settle out in several places, usually the joints and skin, but occasionally in the brain and nerves as well. After two weeks, enough hooks and alarms are around to start combining with them, and an inflammatory reaction starts. The resulting problem ranges from a few aches to a severe arthritis or worse. Most of the time, aspirin or Clinoril® is all that's needed to take care of this. In general, you should use one or the other for this type of arthritis. People often have trouble with joints aching and swelling for some years. Most of the time, this doesn't seem to be due to a lasting infection. Instead, it is related to damage done at the time of the infection. Aspirin or Clinoril® may not always prevent this, but it will probably help. If the reaction becomes more severe, then these drugs should be used to prevent damage to the teflon caps due to poor lubrication. Occasionally the inflammation is so bad that *prednisone* (used every second day) is needed for the short term. If the arthritis lasts a while, the other drugs for RA can also be used.

Some similar things also happen with bacterial infections in the body. Remember that bacteria are little animals that live off the things our body normally uses to feed itself. Bacteria don't grow the way we do—by getting bigger. Instead, they make more of themselves. The body defenses are there to keep this from happening by killing off the bacteria as they are formed. However, sometimes the bacteria can make more of themselves fast enough to overcome the defenses. Most of the time, it's the combination of the bacteria (living or dead) with the hook and alarm assemblies that damages or irritates the joints. This means there has to be a fair number of bugs around somewhere in the body, but not usually in the joints themselves. It also means that the infection must be present for some time to allow time to make lots of hook and alarm assemblies to attach to them. If this hasn't happened, there aren't enough activated alarms to settle out in large numbers in the joints. How long does it take for this type of arthritis to develop? Usually at least two weeks from the start of the infection. More often, several months to a year are required. Our body's defenses are often able to cure the infection within two weeks, and remove it completely. If they can't, the infection becomes quite bad. We then either use antibiotics for it or die. It's the in-between infections, where the body can control the infection but not eliminate it, that cause the joint irritation. This type of infection proceeds slowly, and our body's defenses do their job slowly.

There are quite a number of ways for the bacteria to establish a chronic infection. At one time, *tuberculosis* or TB was a common cause of this. The infection develops slowly and is usually present for some time before it's found and treated. The infection can be in the lung, kidney, throat, intestines, or other areas. As long as enough hooks have been made, these and the breakdown products of the dead bacteria can combine and settle in the joints, causing arthritis. TB, however, can also infect the joints directly, usually in the hip, big toe, or spine.

In women, a relatively common infection that can cause arthritis is a pelvic infection in or near one of the female reproductive organs. These infections can start "on their own," as a result of venereal disease, or following the birth of a child. Sometimes they cause pain. Usually a mild fever 98.8-99.0 is present with a feeling of fatigue and weakness. The fever can be hard to detect especially since the usual glass thermometers won't pick it up. These infections can be very hard to detect since many of the usual tests for infection are normal. The arthritis that results is usually fairly mild with mostly joint stiffness and little swelling. The treatment, of course, is antibiotics for the infection. Sometimes a combination of several must be used. Large amounts for a long period of time are needed, usually several weeks at least. Sometimes treatment is begun with a week's use of antibiotics by vein. Surgery is usually not needed or desirable.

Another likely spot for chronic infections is the intestines. Many parasites will cause infections here, but since they don't release anything that enters the rest of the body, they don't usually cause joint problems. However, there are several chronic infections of the intestine with bacteria that go on for years or decades. These can cause an arthritis that is anything from mild to very severe. The main thing these infections do is to injure the intestine. The intestine is really like a sponge that soaks up the good stuff from the food we eat, puts it into the blood, and passes the rest on along and out. Damage to this sponge prevents the good part of the food from getting into our blood, and therefore the rest of our body. As a result, over a period of years, our body runs short of essential minerals, vitamins and fats while protein and sugar usually get in fine. Over the long run, the bones can become thin from a lack of calcium, and there may be problems with diarrhea or cramping that comes and goes. The problem in the intestine, which is a tube 20 feet long, is worse in some areas. As a result, most people with these infections have some problems getting some things in, but not problems with everything. In addition, there may be a problem with one particular type of sugar—milk sugar or lactose. Some people who have had their intestines damaged by chronic infection develop diarrhea and cramping as an adult whenever they eat anything made with milk. (Incidentally, there is a different type of problem with milk sugar that isn't due to infection. Some people have an intestine that cannot assimilate milk sugar due to hereditary factors. When milk is ingested, these persons react with intestinal cramping and diarrhea but do not contract skin problems. This reaction sometimes begins at birth but more often occurs during late childhood or early adulthood. LactAid® added to the milk or milk product prevents the diarrhea and cramping.

This general type of illness—where food isn't taken into the blood well—is called *maladsorption* (poor intake) or *sprue*. There are other causes of *sprue* besides chronic infection, but they aren't as common. The most common of them is allergy to wheat flour.

Sprue can cause two types of arthritis. The first is from the remains of the intestinal bacteria and the body's hook and alarm assemblies attaching to the lining of the joints. This primarily affects the large joints: knees, hips, wrist, elbows, and fingers. It resembles RA except the wrists aren't involved as much. With *sprue*, the bones don't have as much marble as they should due to poor intake of calcium and other minerals. As a result, the electrical forces in the bones are weak, causing arthritis to develop in the other joints just as in wear and tear arthritis. The fingers, toes, and back in particular are affected. On the other side of the coin, one question to ask if you have wear arthritis at an early age (under 50) is if you're absorbing minerals from your intestine properly. If you have diarrhea frequently, or can't eat milk products, think seriously about sprue as a cause of both problems.

When sprue is due to bacteria, the treatment is a very long term use of antibiotics. Probably either Tagamet® or levamisole should be used in addition. The antibiotic usually prescribed is tetracyline. Because of cost, most people use plain tetracycline, but this can't be taken with milk. Two related and effective antibiotics, doxycycline and minocycline, can be taken with milk. As I mentioned, not all sprue is due to bacteria, but if arthritis is present, it usually is. In some people the diarrhea and cramping aren't even noticeable, and the sprue can only be detected through blood tests. The bacteria can't be grown artificially, or "cultured" as the term goes. If they can be seen in a chunk of the intestine, the disease is called "Whipple's disease." If not, then it's just plain sprue.

For the arthritis itself, usually Clinoril® is best as a treatment until the infection is controlled. Aspirin is OK, too. If this doesn't control the arthritis, first of all the diagnosis should be questioned. Then, the other drugs used for rheumatoid arthritis may be used, if the arthritis is in the large joints. If it is in the small ones—foot, hand, and back, then it's treated like wear arthritis. Cortisone and related drugs (prednisone) should not be used, even as joint injections.

In the types of intestinal infection that cause sprue and Whipple's disease, there isn't any severe permanent damage or scarring to the intestine itself. Once the intestine is cured by antibiotics for a year or two, the intestine is pretty much back to normal. A different type of intestinal infection that can also cause arthritis works a different way. Infection with a completely different type of bacteria causes a great deal of scarring and gradually renders sections of the intestine useless. This infection, like sprue, usually involves most of the intestine at once with some parts hit worse than others. This type of infection also causes diarrhea and a great deal of cramping. The scarred areas break open and pockets of infection, through a leak of the intestines into the belly, also begin. The infection is called Crohn's disease or *regional enteritis* (intestinal inflammation). It's called regional only because one section or another looks bad at a time, even though the problem usually involves the entire intestine at once. The evidence that this disease is due to an infection is quite new and not complete. The bugs haven't been completely identified yet, and what antibiotics, if there are any, that they're sensitive to isn't yet known. Two types of arthritis can occur in this disease. The first comes before the intestinal problem most of the time, and looks like a mild "fusion arthritis" which is discussed later in this chapter. This type of arthritis may not actually be caused by the intestinal infection. The second is due to break-down products of the bacteria causing the infection and the bacteria normally in the intestine that get into the blood from the intestinal damage. These break-down products combine with the hooks formed against them. The arthritis that results for some looks very much like the one in *sprue*. The treatment is the same. If the intestinal disease can be controlled, the arthritis of this second type subsides. The arthritis that resembles fusion arthritis goes its own way, independent of the intestine's problems.

Why do only some of us get these infections? Part of it seems related to which bugs we encounter, but most of it seems to result from what types of hooks we make for the alarms. Some of us, for genetic reasons, don't make very good hooks to latch onto these bugs. If that happens and we come in contact with the bugs, the body's defenses can keep the infection partially in check, but can't cure it.

So far, forms of inflammatory arthritis discussed have been the result of infection elsewhere in the body, but that isn't the only cause of this general type of arthritis. Your body can also react against things that aren't infections. The hook and alarm assemblies, once they're activated, still settle out in the blood vessels and cause inflammation. Anything that gets into the blood that can activate the hook and alarm assemblies does this. It seldom happens because our body is pretty good at screening things from the blood in the first place. In fact, this is what allergies, like hay fever, do. These are a reaction the body has against something that is outside of it, to keep it that way. This, in turn, prevents hooks from being made to attach to these foreign things—dust, plant pollen, etc.—which would set up a more serious inflammatory reaction. People who don't have hay fever can get a special type of arthritis because they don't have an allergy that they really should have. A number of people, either because of their job, hobbies, or just bad luck, breathe in stuff that their body makes hooks against. When this stuff enters the lungs in the absence of hay fever it will go straight into the blood and, from there, to the rest of the body. An allergy would stop this from happening and wash the stuff away. Once hooks have been made against the stuff coming in, a great deal of damage is done in the lungs themselves as the next batch of material enters. However, a good deal of it usually escapes the lungs and goes to the joints. A fairly severe arthritis results as well. The lung problems and the arthritis come on from 4 to 8 hours after exposure to the material at fault, and both last from 8 to 36 hours. A fever and shortness of breath usually accompanies this. The joints may swell and turn red, but usually don't receive permanent damage. There are a whole host of things that can cause this in people who don't have allergies, but common ones are straw, mold in air conditioner filters and humidifiers, animal fur and "dander," pigeon droppings, feathers, and many plant fibers. The gas in silos will cause it, as will some of the chemicals used to make plastics, like polyurethane foam.

However, the various "natural" plant and animal items are the main causes.

There are two other inflammatory diseases that cause arthritis, but, as far as we can tell, are not infections. Both of these diseases cause the same types of arthritis. Each disease can cause two different kinds of arthritis. The first of these diseases is called *psoriasis*, which is a skin problem where scales or flakes are produced on the surface of the skin that come off easily and leave bleeding spots behind. Skin normally has a scale layer at the surface that is very fine and thin. In this disease, too much of this scale is produced too quickly, and usually only on certain parts of the body. The second disease is *ulcerative colitis*. In this disease, the lining of the colon (the large intestine, or last 6 feet of the gut) is being destroyed by the body, for reasons that we really don't understand. Both of these diseases can produce an arthritis that looks just like RA, with pain and swelling in the large joints—the knee, hip, elbow, shoulder, wrist, and at the bases of the toes and fingers—that comes and goes. Usually there is little if any actual destruction of the joints. The disease operates exactly like RA. Hooks and alarms combine with material from the skin or colon while the blood passes through these parts of the body. If not all the attached hook and alarm assemblies are removed from the blood before they reach the joints, they settle out there, already activated. They then trigger the destruction of the stuff they've attached to, and the blood vessels and lining of the joints are injured as an innocent bystander.

The second type of arthritis these diseases can cause involves the joints in the pelvis (which have no lining at all) and the fingers and toes. Occasionally the bones of the spine may also be involved, causing the growth of large spurs that fuse the bones together, across the flexible hinges. This type of arthritis seems to be the result of the production of hooks and alarms during the course of the *psoriasis* or *colitis* that react mistakenly with the teflon in the joints of the fingers and the cement that holds the joints of the pelvis together. These joints are then directly attacked, since the alarms are on them and triggered by the attachment of the hooks. The problem in this type of arthritis seems to be a failure of the suppressor cells. They should prevent the production of these hooks that attach to the joint themselves, but apparently they don't recognize that wrong ones are being made. This type of arthritis is usually mild in these diseases. In psoriasis, though, it can be particularly severe and destroy the joints of the hands and feet.

The treatment of these forms of arthritis is similar to that for RA, although aspirin works poorly, and is often not worth trying. Treatments that help the *psoriasis* will also help the arthritis, and some of the newer treatments (*psoralen,* dialysis, *methotrexate*) that work for psoriasis may be desirable if the arthritis is severe. Gold injections are often effective. Plaquanil® generally should not be used since it may make the psoriasis worse. *Penacillamine* and *auranofin* also run this risk, but less is known about the actual dangers involved. *Levamisole* and Tagamet®, because of their ability to stimulate the suppressor cells, may prove useful for both of these forms of arthritis in both diseases. Preliminary evidence indicates that Tagamet® is also an effective treatment for some forms of psoriasis. When the severe and rapidly destructive form of arthritis is present in *psoriasis*, it may be necessary to proceed directly with *methotrexate*, Cytoxan®, or *prednisone* to preserve the joints, and add other treatments later.

Before ending discussion of these diseases, there are three important things to remember: First, not all colitis is *ulcerative colitis*. This latter form is relatively rare. If you've been told you have colitis, don't assume that you have this type, unless you've been told specifically that you do. Second, not everyone with these two diseases gets the arthritis. Usually the liver and spleen can filter out the activated alarms from the blood and prevent it. Third, if you have *psoriasis* and arthritis, there is a joint infection, called Reiter's disease, that causes a skin problem identical to a severe form of *psoriasis* and an arthritis very similar to that seen with real *psoriasis*. Unlike *psoriasis*, this disease has a cure and is important to recognize. It's discussed later in this chapter.

One of the types of arthritis occurring with *psoriasis* and colitis is different from the other inflammatory types of arthritis. The joint surfaces themselves were what the hooks were directed against. There are three other types of arthritis where the joint surfaces are attacked directly. The first of these is joint infections, where bacteria attack the joint by multiplying inside it; these infections aren't discussed in this book. In the other two, the body itself is directing an attack on the teflon cap in the joints.

In the first of these, the arthritis is most severe in the joints of the pelvis, which normally have no movement at all, and in the flexible hinges between the bones of the spine. Again, there is no movement of these bones against each other, at least not in the way the hips or knees move. As this type of arthritis progresses, the joints fuse together with bridges of solid bone. In the pelvis this doesn't cause a serious problem, besides pain as the arthritis progresses. In the spine, however, the freezing can cause real difficulty. In the most severe situation, a person can no longer bend, turn, take a deep breath, or twist. This arthritis, which I think we should call fusion arthritis, has the medical name *ankylosing spondylitis,* which means fusion of the surfaces of the bones.

Fusion arthritis usually begins between 12 and 15 years of age. It affects men and women equally (contrary to the belief of many physicians) but may be milder and harder to recognize in women. The ability to get the arthritis is inherited, although the arthritis itself is not. The first thing a person usually feels is pain low in the back on both sides. The pain increases with twisting and bending. This represents the start of the arthritis in the joints of the pelvis, which are always the first ones involved. The next place for the arthritis to show up is in the spine, at the area of the chest and the lower back. The neck area is usually involved later. At first, there's pain and stiffness with turning and bending. If the chest is seriously involved, there is also pain in deep breathing. As the arthritis progresses, the bones of the lower back and, later, the chest freeze together. The joint between the collarbone and the shoulder, and between the collarbone and the central bones of the chest may also be affected. In addition, a mild arthritis, with occasional joint swelling, pain, and stiffness, can start in the hips, knees, shoulders, and ankles. Most of the problem here is usually stiffness, but with some people, the arthritis at these places can be severe.

At one time physicians claimed this type of arthritis was rare. Recently, some have claimed it affects 5% of the population. The truth probably is that 5% are susceptible, but far fewer get it. The basic problem seems to be the development of hook and alarm assemblies that attach to the teflon caps on the bones that have motionless joints or flexible hinges. The attack is initially at the place where the cables that hold the joints together are anchored, at the edge of the caps. The teflon the body uses for these joints is chemically a bit different from that in the other joints, so it's relatively easy for the body to make a hook that will attach well to one and poorly to the other. Chemical similarities between the teflons account for the fact that sometimes in fusion arthritis, the hips, knees, and other joints may also be involved. Once the hooks attach to the teflon of these joints, the teflon is attacked by the detergents that the alarms activate. The white blood cells are attracted by this activated detergent and give off chemicals that make blood vessels grow around the joint and into it. The pain comes from the P-G's and other chemicals released from the bone as these blood vessels grow in. This stimulates new bone to form over the new blood vessels. The bone that's laid down fuses the joints. In the spine, the bood vessels, and therefore the

FUSION ARTHRITIS

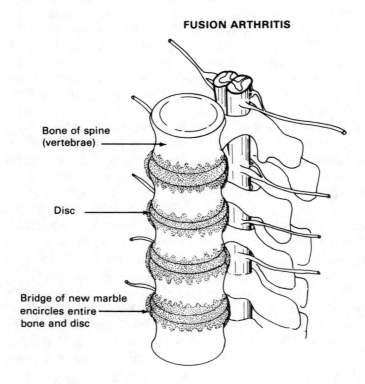

Bone of spine (vertebrae)

Disc

Bridge of new marble encircles entire bone and disc

bone, are laid down along the line of the flexible hinges, or discs, that connect the bones together. This happens all the way around the disc, both above and below. When the marble growing down meets the stuff coming up, the bones fuse together.

What causes this disease? Right now there is no good answer, but there are clues. Part of the problem lies in the suppressor cells. They fail to stop the production of hooks that attach to the teflon of these joints. Since their abilities are hereditary, this explains in part the hereditary factor in this disease. But not everyone who can get the arthritis does indeed get it. Something people are exposed to in their surroundings must play a role; the first thought is an infection.

How do you treat this type of arthritis and can it be stopped? Currently, the main emphasis in treatment is the use of drugs to stop or slow its progression. There are none that reverse it. All drugs commonly used for this purpose seem to work by inhibiting production of the P-G's. This both decreases pain and decreases the growth of the new blood vessels that cause the bone fusion. Aspirin does not work well, however, and is not even worth trying. The most effective drug for this disease is Clinoril®. Depending on the severity of the disease, and how fast it is progressing, the dosage is from 150 mg once a day to 600 mg twice a day. In general, it's wise to take at least 150 mg a day as a minimum, since the drug is used both to give comfort and slow the course of the illness. If Clinoril® has too many undesired effects, the replacements for it discussed in the next chapter can be used. The next-best drug is Indocin.®.

For people with extremely rapid disease progression, prednisone may be needed. In any event, remember that these drugs do not change the underlying cause of the disease, nor will they help a joint that has already fused or been destroyed.

The usual other drugs for RA, like the gold drugs, penacillamine, Plaquanil® in particular, are not usually effctive for this type of arthritis although they may be of help if the hip is involved. No information is available in this regard for auranofin and Cytoxan®, though auranofin may be very successful in this disease. The drugs that stimulate the suppressor cells work well in preliminary trials. *Levamisole*, again, has been the main one used and is fairly effective. Tagamet® has had much less use and its true effectiveness for fusion arthritis isn't yet known. When *levamisole* becomes available, it may become the best treatment for this disease.

The tendency for bony fusion to take place in this disease makes several simple things important. Most of them relate to the back. Since, despite the above treatments, there is a real possibility that some or all of the bones in the back may fuse, it's important to keep these bones in straight alignment. That way, when and if they do fuse, you aren't left bent over double or unable to breathe. Consequently, it's important to sleep on a very hard mattress, without a pillow or with a very low (1-2") one at the most. Always sit straight in firm, straight-backed chairs. Sit with good posture as well. Exercises that keep the back as limber as possible are important, as well as those that keep the hips and shoulders moving. Many physicians recommend swimming. Tennis, golf, and manual work that involves lots of bending aren't the best, since even people without this type of arthritis tend to get spurs in the back from this. The exercises in the section on wear arthritis can be used for the shoulders and hips to keep them limber.

The greatest damage in fusion arthritis usually occurs in the spine. Once it is fused, little can be done. For the most severe situations, when a person is bent over double, the bones in the spine can be cut apart and repositioned. However, this is an extremely dangerous operation, and is used only in the most severe situations. Occasionally the hip is severely involved and, in that circumstance, it can and should be replaced, even in young people. There are three points of caution in fusion arthritis. Occasionally eye involvement can occur, requiring application of *prednisone*-like drugs to the eye. Second, this arthritis is often mistakenly called RA or just "back trouble." Third, occasionally Reiter's disease is called fusion arthritis by mistake. Since Reiter's disease has a special cure, this isn't a good mistake to make. So, if you've been told you have fusion arthritis, look at the section on Reiter's disease later in this chapter, as well as the section on the arthritis that accompanies *psoriasis* and intestinal disorders, earlier in this chapter.

There is a second type of arthritis in which the body tries to destroy the teflon caps in the joints. This is much less common than fusion arthritis, and tends to happen at most any age. The teflon that is attacked makes up most of the joints that move, like the knees, hips, fingers, and such. This type of teflon, however, is also the same stuff that makes up the "skeleton" of the ear and nose, and the front portion of the ribs. Since many teflon (or cartilage) areas are attacked, the disease is called *polychondritis*. One odd characteristic of this disease is that it comes and goes, and there may be problem-free periods when nothing seems to go wrong.

In *polychondritis*, hook and alarm assemblies are partially involved in attacking the teflon but much of the destruction is done by white blood cells with hooks attached. Any place with this teflon can be attacked. The arthritis looks very much like RA, and the only thing that tips you off that it isn't RA is the fact that the ear, front of the chest, or nose are involved. Presumably, the problem again is in the suppressor cells. The initial event is probably an infection somewhere in the body. Once the body starts making hooks against itself, the teflon will cause the hooks to be continually produced, unless the suppressor cells stop it. Occasionally, *polychondritis* is part of an arthritis that is obviously due to an infection, as discussed in the first part of this chapter. In that case, sometimes fluid-filled blisters are present in the skin, or red streaks appear as a tip-off to the actual presence of the infection.

The usual treatment to date has been *prednisone* and drugs like Clinoril®. Preferably, as discussed in the next chapter, the *prednisone* is used every second day. The nature of the infection that sets off this disease usually isn't known. This illness seems like the ideal place for the white blood cell stimulating drugs, like *levamisole* and Tagamet®. To date, not much use has been made of these drugs. However, there has been some success with Tagamet®. Other drugs for RA, like *penacillamine*, Plaquanil®, and particularly *auranofin,* should be of use, but there hasn't been much experience with them, either. The white blood cell supressants, like Cytoxan® will also work but these drugs are undesirable due to the dangers of use, and are reserved only for use against rapid joint destruction. In general *auranofin* and *levamisole*/Tagamet® are preferred as treatment.

Since the spine isn't affected, the exercises and other measures for fusion arthritis aren't of use. The illness is really one of direct destruction of the teflon cap, without fusion. Once the teflon at the ends of the bones is destroyed, however, the joint can fuse together. The main exercise-related thing is to avoid hurting the joints that are involved. The damage to the teflon caps means that great care for the affected joints is very important, until the medications can control the destruction and let the teflon be repaired. Any exercise that stresses an irritated joint should be cut. For example, if a knee is affected, avoid running and climbing completely, and stand as little as possible. If the nose is affected, don't get bumped on the nose.

The severity and speed with which the joint destruction can progress makes it a good idea to start treatment with *prednisone* (or *levamisole*/Tagamet®) and Clinoril®, and add in other drugs like *auranofin* and Plaquanil®. After the latter start to work, a few days to a few weeks later, the *prednisone* can be stopped or reduced. Since the disease lasts a long time and tends to come back again, it usually pays to use one or more of the other drugs rather than go through the difficulties of the long-term use of *prednisone*.

Several times in this chapter, I've mentioned a joint infection called Reiter's disease. This illness came up because of its surprising similarities with the arthritis of *psoriasis*, intestinal disease, and fusion arthritis. Now it's time for the details about Reiter's disease.

Reiter's disease is pretty much a problem of adults, and usually starts some time after 18. A few instances of fusion arthritis and RA or juvenile RA in children may actually be Reiter's disease, appearing at an early age. It happens about equally often in men and women, but is rarely recognized in women, so that it appears to be much more common in men. It is far more severe when it occurs in people who have the genetic susceptibility to fusion arthritis. This susceptibility can be determined with a blood test.

The first thing that the bugs which cause Reiter's disease do is to cause diarrhea or just stomach cramps. The arthritis appears only later, often after the appearance of burning with urination, dry irritated eyes, or severe *psoriasis* (scaling skin) of the feet and hands in particular. The arthritis appears to be caused by the same bacteria that caused the diarrhea and other problems, after they have lost their outer coating or cell wall, and have started to live within the body's own cells. The early problems in Reiter's disease may be so mild that they go unnoticed, compared to the arthritis that can follow.

The arthritis is present day after day, as well as creating sudden attacks of pain and swelling. Usually the joints lowest down on the body are the most affected. The toes, feet, and ankles generally tend to be much worse than the knees, hips and arm joints, though this isn't always the case. Unlike RA, the joints in the pelvis are often involved as well. Unlike fusion arthritis, one side is usually much worse than the other, while in fusion arthritis, both sides are equally bad. An x-ray of these joints sometimes doesn't show the arthritis in these last joints, and a special test, called a technecium scan, sometimes is needed to show the arthritis in the pelvic bones. This type of arthritis, if not treated with the proper antibiotics, progresses throughout a person's life, with only a very rare person "curing himself." It can progress at a different rate in different people, and at times may seem to be at a standstill for a few months. In the long run, though, it may lead to severe joint destruction in many people. Usually the features mentioned above allow you to differentiate Reiter's disease from fusion arthritis and the other similar problems. If there's still doubt about what the real problem is, the level of the body's antibacterial detergent in the joint fluid can be measured. It's usually quite high in Reiter's disease, and normal or low in the others.

What do you do about this form of arthritis? To ease the pain and keep the joint destruction in check while the disease is being treated with antibiotics, Clinoril® is the best drug to use. Aspirin works poorly and is not worth trying. If Clinoril® can't be used, again see the next chapter for alternatives. Plaquanil® and the gold-containing drugs (particularly *auranofin*) can help the arthritis. However, if the skin problems are also present, they can become much worse with these drugs (except perhaps *auranofin*), and may have to be avoided for this reason. If *prednisone* is used for arthritis, its use should be brief, and if possible, every second day. Tagamet® and *levamisole* can be very useful drugs, both for relieving the arthritis, and for helping to cure the infection. However, since they increase the white blood cells' reaction to the infection, they may make the pain and abdominal cramping much worse at first, and you may have to wait until antibiotics have been used a while to start them.

What antibiotics do you use? For bacteria that live within the body's cells, only a few can be used. Usually the tetracycline-type is best, but it has to be used without interruption for 6-18 months to cure it. Occasionally 2 years are needed. That's a long time, but considering the outcome of this disease without the treatment, it's really worth it. Remember that the antibiotic can't reverse the damage that has been done to the joints, so it's important to start it promptly. If a person is allergic to *tetracycline*, there are two related antibiotics that don't usually have the allergy problems and might be worth a try: *doxycycline* and *minocycline*. Otherwise, there are a few other antibiotics for this general type of bacteria: *chloramphenicol*, Septra® and Cleocin®. In general they are much less desirable for use. As mentioned above, along with the antibiotics, a white blood cell stimulating drug, like Tagamet®, may be a good idea.

While the arthritis is being treated, it is important to put as little stress on the involved joints as possible. This means limited walking, no running, and lots of sitting. The involved joints should be put through exercises that take them through their full range of motion at least once a day, to prevent their fusing together. Since the spine is involved in Reiter's disease, as in fusion arthritis, people with Reiter's under treatment should take the same precautions as outlined for people with fusion arthritis earlier in this chapter.

The overlap between Reiter's disease, fusion arthritis, and the other similar types of arthritis I've mentioned earlier is striking. It seems certain that there's some basic connection between these diseases, even though they seem to have different causes. What it is just isn't clear yet. But it does seem to be more than just the inheritable "genetic susceptibility" for fusion arthritis mentioned earlier. Most likely, it's related to what the white blood cells can and can't react against.

Look-Alikes for Rheumatoid Arthritis

A number of diseases that aren't basically a form of arthritis can cause stiffness or joint pain in a way that makes them look like RA. Since these diseases have different treatments and outlooks as to what will happen to your body, they're worth knowing about. All the diseases in this last section are frequently called RA by mistake. If you've been told you have RA, it would be worth your while to look at this section.

As in RA itself, part of what goes wrong in these diseases involves a mistake on the part of the suppressor white blood cells, discussed in the previous chapter. In all these illnesses, hook and alarm assemblies are made that attach to normal parts of the body, or the seek-and-destroy white blood cells have hooks attached that accomplish the same thing. In each of these diseases, an infection that the body can't get rid of probably caused the hooks to be made in the first place. It is usually a virus, although in one of these diseases it may be a special type of bacteria. At this point you may want to go back and look over the first part of the chapter on RA that goes into the hooks and alarms, and the white blood cells. For review, I'll go over the story very quickly.

When things the body doesn't want to have around—like infections with bacteria and viruses—get into our body, it produces special tags that attach to each separate thing that shouldn't be there and pinpoints it for destruction. The tags are really tiny hooks that latch on to special areas on the surface of a bacteria or virus. They won't stick just anywhere. Some of these hooks are at the end of a cord that has an "alarm" or signal on the other hand. This signal pulls in and activates detergents that are in our blood to destroy the tagged invader. Other hooks are attached to white blood cells. Hook attachment activates the cell and causes it to destroy the invader on the other end of the hook. Normally, hooks can only be made against things that are not naturally in our body. If a mistake is made and a hook is produced against something that really should be there, a special type of white blood cell called a suppressor cell seeks out the source of the hooks and stops it from working. A number of diseases, among them RA, are partially the result of a lapse in the surveillance of these suppressor cells. These hooks that attach to the normal parts of the body are made by mistake. The body is actually trying to make hooks that will attach to viruses or bacteria that are causing an infection, but some people can't make hooks that attach properly to certain types of bacteria or viruses. As a result, the infection lasts a long time, and is difficult to get rid of. The continued presence of this infection usually stimulates the white blood cells to make more and more hooks. Since these hooks aren't very accurate or particular and also attach to the normal parts of the body, as long as the infection is present more hooks are made that end up doing more harm than good.

Why don't these hooks, even though they aren't the best, eventually get rid of the infection? If it were just a matter of making more hooks, the job would be easy. In fact, in most of these illnesses, a tremendous number of hooks are made, but the problem isn't one of numbers. It's one of hideouts. In the chronic infections that cause the diseases in this section, the viruses and bacteria are actually hiding in the body's cells. They aren't so easy to get at. It's like the wolf who attacks a herd of sheep by covering himself with a lamb's skin, except these wolves are even smarter: they actually live inside a sheep without killing it! To get rid of this type of infection, the hooks must be extremely well-made and accurate.

When bacteria live in our cells, they still keep their own form and remain a single unit. They always have some sort of barrier that separates them from the cell they're living in. Once inside our cells, they open little holes in the barrier so the food and stuff inside our cells can go into the bacteria as well. The barrier, however, can still be recognized by some of our white blood cells as "foreign." Since these white blood cells can also get inside our own body's cells, these bacteria can still be destroyed by them. Antibiotics can also poison these bacteria even though they're inside our cells. The hook and alarm assemblies, as far as we know, can't go into our cells. They can only get the bugs when they come out of the cells to go into the blood.

When the viruses go into hiding, they are much sneakier than the bacteria. The bacteria, even when in hiding, can exist only as an intact package; the whole bug has to be there. The viruses, on the other hand, can exist with one piece here and another piece somewhere else since the viruses are basically two parts. There is an outer wrapper, or envelope, and an inner piece of "magnetic tape" that carries the code for making more viruses. It's usually the outer wrapper that the body recognizes as foreign, and makes hooks against it. When a virus infects one of the cells of our body, only the code goes in. The wrapper is left behind on the outside. The code then takes over our cell's machinery and tells it to make wrappers and more code strips. These usually are combined and released. When the virus goes into hiding, it simply remains in the cell as a code only. Few or no wrappers are made and released. The virus, as a code alone, stays on inside the cell. Usually, in this situation, a few wrappers are made and assembled with the code strip, but the number is very few. And if these few are released, the cell usually is not destroyed in the process. When the virus code strip remains in the cell without telling it to make many new viruses and release them, the code strip can do several things. It may just float around free, and use the cell's machinery from time to time. It can also join in with our own code strips and actually become part of our genetic code. In that case, it literally takes up permanent residence.

What does our body do when the virus goes into hiding? Sometimes it doesn't have to do anything if the virus just sits there and doesn't do anything. But there are several important defenses our body has against viruses in hiding. The first centers around the fact that most viruses in hiding still release a few complete viruses into the blood now and then. When the white blood cells find them, they release a special chemical that tells other cells to look for pieces of the virus code inside them, and if they find it, to break it down and not make more of it. Another defense centers around the virus code telling the cell to make things that are not normally in the cells—the parts that go into the virus envelope and code. These things are not made into new viruses, but do end up on the surface of the cell in our body. Once they are on the surface, both the hooks and alarms in the blood, and the white blood cells with hooks attached, can recognize these cells as different from what they should be. They are coated, lightly, with stuff that shouldn't be there and these cells are destroyed, along with the virus in them.

This system works well most of the time. If the virus sits there and does nothing, it doesn't matter if it's there or not. If our body can destroy all the cells that contain the virus, again that's OK. One or another of these things is what happens most of the time. But with a system like this, there's room for a real problem. Remember that what we make hooks against is determined by our heredity. If we're unlucky and we have trouble making good hooks against these viruses, then we don't have alarms that can trigger the destruction of the cells that contain the viruses. Also, our white blood cells (which use the same hooks) can't recognize these cells. As a result, our body can keep the virus only partially under control, and has to rely on the first defense system, discussed above. Then we have a virus infection that isn't completely suppressed. Some of the viruses or their parts (envelopes or code strips) are constantly being placed on the surface of cells and released into our blood. We are constantly making more and more hooks in an attempt to cure ourselves. Sometimes, these hooks will react with our own bodies as well, either because of a mistake in the production of hooks, or because the virus has changed the surface of many of the cells in our body by putting parts of its envelope or code out there. As a result, the body may be constantly trying to get rid of a virus, and have a chronic inflammatory disease. What form it takes depends on several things: Where the virus is in the body; how well the hooks and alarms, once activated, are trapped in the liver and spleen; and how good the suppressor white blood cells are at keeping the body from reacting against itself.

Before I tell you about these diseases in particular and what to look for, I should point out that they can be inherited. Sometimes it's the virus that's inherited, sometimes the limitations on what hooks can be made. But there's another thing. To destroy the cells containing the viruses, the hooks and alarms need to activate a detergent system in the blood and body fluids. If there is a problem with this system, even if everything else is normal, a chronic virus infection can result. Problems with this detergent system are also inherited. Having this type of problem passed down the line in a family will also cause each person to have a chronic virus infection if they are exposed to a virus that can cause this.

At this time it looks as if all the diseases in this last section that are look-alikes for RA are chronic infections, probably viral. The first one, called *lupus* (yes, the name does mean wolf) can be the hardest to distinguish from RA.

Lupus most often starts in younger women (25-40 years) but can occur at any age in either men or women, as well as in children. It causes joint aching, stiffness, and swelling in the same joints involved by RA. The thing that makes it different is that the problems tend to come and go frequently, rather than coming and staying. The actual amount of joint damage is usually minimal for the amount of pain and discomfort experienced. The other thing about *lupus* is that much more than the joints are involved. Often a skin rash, large lymph nodes, fever, serious changes in the blood count, and kidney problems are present as well. Some of these things you won't see yourself, especially the last two which require special tests. Your doctor will generally check these things as a matter of course. In addition, *lupus* will often cause problems with the nerves in the arms, legs, or brain. Other common things involved in *lupus* are the lungs, making it painful to breathe, and the heart, causing chest pain or shortness of breath. All of these symptoms will frequently get better and worse as time goes on.

The thing that visibly sets *lupus* apart from RA is the many things that go wrong. Not everyone with *lupus* has all these things happen, but virtually everyone has more than just joint problems as a result. This makes it relatively easy to tell the two apart. All this happens in *lupus* because the code from the virus at fault is actually released into the blood, as well as being on the cell surfaces. It combines with hook and alarm assemblies in many spots in the body. Most likely, cells in many parts of the body harbour the virus, and are constantly being destroyed by both the hook and alarm assemblies and the white blood cells as well.

Another disease that is mistaken for RA surprisingly

often is an inflammatory disease of muscle, called *polymyositis* (many muscle inflammation). This disease can feel like RA because the arms and legs, hips, and often the back can be quite sore and painful. In addition, the skin over the knees and ankles can pick up a blue-violet color. As in RA, the arms and legs hurt much more when moving and working, and there may be severe morning stiffness. The real differences are that it's the muscles that hurt, and weakness is usually more of a problem than pain, though not always. The joints never actually swell. *Polymyositis* doesn't involve free hook and alarm assemblies. In this disease, the white blood cells with attached hooks do the damage. Again, this illness appears to be the result of a persistent virus in the muscles. However, unlike *lupus*, the virus seems to be limited to the muscles, or occasionally muscles and skin. No partial viruses are released into the blood, so no activated hook and alarm assemblies are around to settle out in the joints.

Lupus and *polymyositis* are two extremes of a situation. With *lupus*, most of the damage is the result of viral codes circulating and reacting with hook and alarm assemblies in the body. In *polymyositis*, the code never makes it out of the cells. The attack is made by the white blood cells, alone, and is probably brought on by a virus-caused change in the surface of the cells.

There is a third disease that is a variation of *lupus*. It comes about for a very special reason. There are two large families of viruses in this world. They're different because their genetic codes are made from different types of our cells to make something, the instructions are rewritten letters called DNA. When the library needs to be used by our cells to make soemthing, the instructions are rewritten in a second alphabet called RNA. The alphabets are similar, but for each letter there's a distinct difference, like the difference between roman and *italic* letters.

Like ourselves, many viruses have their library of codes

written in DNA. The viruses that cause *lupus* seem to do this, too, since the codes floating in the blood are DNA. If a DNA-coded virus can cause *lupus*, why can't a virus that uses RNA do the same thing? Well, they almost can. There are many viruses that have their code written in RNA. They can also establish chronic infections. But the disease they cause is somewhat different, and is given a different name. There's no common name for it yet, but the medical name is *mixed connective tissue disease*. Connective tissue is the stuff that ties things together: muscles, ligaments, skin, etc. For simplicity, let's call it RNA-lupus. The way this disease occurs is basically the same as *lupus* but the problems it causes are different, and it's not clear why. The main features of this disease are, first of all, an arthritis that is usually similar to *lupus*. It comes and goes with a good deal of stiffness and aching, and some swelling. Usually, there is no joint destruction and all in all, the arthritis is mild. However, some people with RNA-lupus have fairly severe arthritis with a great deal of swelling and joint destruction. Then the arthritis looks identical to RA, and can be every bit as severe. In all cases, other things are present as well, just as with *lupus*. Often, a problem called Raynaud's disease is present. In this, the blood vessels in the fingers, and sometimes the toes, narrow off when they are exposed to cold or irritation. This shuts off the blood supply in the fingers and makes them turn sheet-white and numb. Sometimes the skin becomes swollen, and later very thin. Little hard lumps can form in the skin in areas where painful red spots had appeared earlier. There may be a sense of tightness in the throat and trouble swallowing as the muscle in the tube from the mouth to the stomach is damaged. The skin, especially of the face and hands, gets red, spidery marks on it and the fingers and face lose their creases and folds with partial loss of the fingerprints. Usually a muscle problem that looks identical to *polymy-*

ositis is present, although its cause is different. There are special blood tests to help diagnose this illness. Much of the treatment is similar to RA, although *prednisone* is often necessary for features other than the arthritis. If the hard lumps in the skin are especially a problem (they are made of calcium—bone marble), sometimes Didronel® is used to prevent their formation.

The last really important look-alike for RA is virtually found only in older people, although on rare occasion it appears in people as young as 40. In this disease, the main problem is tremendous arm, leg, and back stiffness. Like RA, it's more severe in the morning on rising and can be a bit better once you get moving. There may be a bit of fever, too, which is not typical for RA in adults. The pain comes from the muscles and tendons (cables that link the muscles to the bones) and seems to be coming from around the joints. The joints are not tender to the touch, but the muscles may be. One common thing is pain in the face. In particular, the pain is right over the upper set of teeth, on one or both sides, and comes from a large muscle that does the work in chewing. There may also be severe headaches involving one or both temples. The arteries (blood vessels) that run across the temples may be very tender or have a knotty feel. In the most severe form of this disease, there may be temporary or permanent loss of vision in an eye.

The exact cause of this disease isn't clear, but it appears to be an infection, involving either the sheaths covering the muscle tendons alone, or plus the walls of the arteries themselves. When it involves the sheaths alone, it's called *polymyalgia rheumatica* (many muscle aches). Obviously it isn't an arthritis at all. When only the tendons are involved, the jaw pain, headaches, and vision problems are never present. Also, most blood tests and muscle tests are normal, except occasionally the liver shows an irritation. One test, called the sedimentation rate, is always far from normal. When the arteries are also involved, it's called *temporal arteritis* (irritation of the forehead arteries). This appears to be an infection of both the walls of the arteries and the tendon sheaths by something which may or may not be a virus. The headache, jaw pain, and loss of eyesight are due to a closing off of the arteries due to irritation. This is a fairly serious problem, and requires a different treatment than does the *polymyalgia* alone.

Temporal arteritis involves almost all the arteries in the body, not just the ones in the forehead. In fact when it occurs in young people (15-30 years of age) without the tendon problems, it primarily involves the very large arteries off the heart, and usually doesn't affect the ones in the head at all. This variation of the disease, incidentally, is called "pulseless disease" since the pulses are lost in the arms.

At this time, evidence suggests that the infection involved in these diseases isn't a virus, but some other form of life, possibly a bacteria. However, what antibiotic, if any, should be used isn't known. The current treatments are *prednisone* for the arteritis and aspirin for the aches. Probably Clinoril® is better for this purpose, though *auranofin* may eventually prove to be the best treatment. When the arteritis is present, treatment is especially important, since once the arteries close, they won't reopen. Usually this disease ends of its own accord in 2-4 years, which would suggest that the body slowly cures itself of the infection.

Just as *polymyalgia* and *temporal arteritis* can look like forms of arthritis, there are several other diseases that can look like these two. *Polymyositis* can feel and look like *polymyalgia*, as can some forms of cancer in their early stages. Other diseases that injure the arteries, called *vasculitis* (inflammation of the blood vessels) can all look like both *temporal arteritis* and *polymyalgia*, which are really quite different. How do you know when to worry about a mistake along these lines? By the response to treatment. *Polymyalgia* improves a lot and fast with a moderate amount of aspirin or Clinoril®. *Temporal arteritis* gets better fast with *prednisone*. If that isn't the case, chances are that the diagnosis isn't the correct one.

Determining the problem and its treatment

Deciding What's Wrong

OBVIOUSLY, not all types of arthritis are the same. Although treatments are often similar from one type of arthritis to another, there are many differences. These differences are not only in what you can use as a treatment, but in what you can expect from the arthritis in the future. Either way, it's important to determine what type of arthritis is present at the beginning. This section summarizes some of the characteristics of the various types of arthritis to help you decide between them for your own diagnosis of what's wrong. This section is brief, assuming that you have at least read through the "characteristics" summary in each of the previous chapters. (These are listed in the index.)

The first thing in determining what's wrong is to decide whether the problem is arthritis or not. *With arthritis, the pain or swelling is in a joint, not around it.* If you don't feel a joint sitting right where it hurts, the problem may not be arthritis. One exception to this is arthritis in the pelvic joints. These joints don't usually move, and you can't touch them directly. It feels as if the pain is low in the back and not from a joint. These pelvic joints hurt most when walking, since they twist a bit at that time. Remember that there are flexible joints in the back and true joints that "bend" high in the neck, and at the base of the skull where it meets the neck.

Most people think that if the problem is arthritis, there's pain when you move. That's true sometimes, but not always. Particularly in children, but also in adults, there may not be any pain: just stiffness or swelling. That is still arthritis. Pain outside of the joints—in the tendons, ligaments, and their sheaths—isn't arthritis, although in some problems, like rheumatoid arthritis and gout, this often accompanies the arthritis.

Now that you're sure you have arthritis, how do you tell what type it is? The first criterion to use is age. In a younger adult—under 50—wear and tear arthritis is very unusual, although it can happen, particularly in joints that are already damaged by something else. If there are also problems with the areas around the joints—the tendons and ligaments—then gout, RA, and of course the look-alikes for RA are good thoughts. The arthritis of gout comes on suddenly and is very painful. RA, on the other hand, is a more chronic, on-going illness with a more moderate level of pain. Morning stiffness is very prominent in RA, less so in wear arthritis, and even less so in gout. RA tends to involve the small joints of the hand and wrist. Gout usually doesn't involve the hand itself, but will occur at the wrist.

Fusion arthritis usually starts in the late teens or twenties with a pain that feels as if it comes from deep inside or between the hips. Later on, the arthritis of *psoriasis*, Reiter's disease, and intestinal disease can start the same way. The presence of a skin problem or intestinal problem is the signal to consider these other types of arthritis.

In adults, when arthritis is associated with infection, particularly if in the intestines, periodic fevers, abdominal cramps, and diarrhea can occur. On occasion, the joints in the pelvis are also involved. Infections of the joints themselves cause a fairly severe arthritis of just one or occasionally two joints, most often. The big exception to this is gonorrhea, which usually involves many joints at once and is accompanied by a skin rash.

For people over 50, wear and tear arthritis is the major problem. RA can start at ages over 50, but usually it has stopped progressing by that age and now the joints are undergoing accelerated wear and tear. The absence of swelling and the improvement of morning stiffness for someone who has previously had RA usually signals the start of this process. By age 50, fusion arthritis has usually stabilized, except in people who do not have the "genetic susceptibility" to it but got it anyway. The arthritis of psoriasis, or Reiter's disease, can start at this age and look like fusion arthritis on the surface of things. For people over 50, the greatest difficulty is in distinguishing between the look-alikes for RA and wear arthritis. The presence of little bony nodules or spurs around the joints is a fairly good sign that wear arthritis is present. Its look-alikes may also be present, so don't be misled. The thickening of the joint bag's lining that is typical of RA is present in lupus and RNA-lupus, but not in the other look-alikes for RA. The nodules in the skin (rheumatoid nodules) typical of RA won't occur in any of the look-alikes, although RNA-lupus can cause very hard, painful lumps in the skin. Remember, not everyone with RA has the nodules, though.

Occasionally gout will give a first attack after the age of 50 and show up as a joint that is suddenly painful. Just as often at this age a sudden attack of arthritis, even if it's in the big toe, can be due to wear arthritis or pseudogout.

The Treatments: General Principles

One of the really unfortunate things about medicine is that very little good news wanders in out of the blue. New cures and better treatments for any disease, including arthritis, are pretty much the result of long and difficult work. New treatments, in their final form, aren't chance discoveries. That doesn't mean that a lucky break or a chance finding won't occur. They may be the start of something really good, or may speed things along, but by and large, even the lucky break is only the start of a long line of hard work.

One good example of this is aspirin. The 100th anniversary of the lucky discovery of aspirin · was 1978. But it wasn't all luck. In 1870, world supplies of quinine, a drug used for fever, pain, and malaria, were running short. People were looking for something else to use. So, one by one, they made extracts of literally hundreds of plants related to the one quinine comes from until they found a plant whose extract could lower fever. The chemical in the extract responsible for this was aspirin. It took a century of work to learn just what aspirin would do. The discovery of the usefulness of aspirin in the treatment of hardening of the arteries, strokes, and heart attacks comes almost 100 years after the initial discovery of the drug. The full usefulness of aspirin in this regard still isn't known. Most of the drugs used for arthritis today are further developments of aspirin, but these developments took over 50 years of intensive work, and several hundred million dollars.

Most of what is coming in the next ten years for arthritis is a fairly logical development of what's available now. With the current FDA controls on drugs and treatments, even if something totally unexpected were discovered, the marketing of the discovery would be about 10 years away after all tests for safety and effectiveness were completed.

When a drug is approved by the FDA, the approval comes only after extensive testing for both effectiveness and safety in people with the disease being treated. It isn't possible to have a perfectly safe drug that is completely effective. All approvals are a judgment by the FDA that tries to balance off the good and the bad. Drugs for minor problems, like colds and coughs, have to be very safe before they are released because the problem being treated isn't too serious. Drugs for the treatment of advanced cancer by and large have many ill effects that are expected from their use. Since the disease these drugs treat is so terrible, their use is reasonable. Most drugs, of course, are in between the two extremes. Only the safest drugs are released for use without a doctor's advice; that is, for sale over the counter. When the FDA releases a drug, the release is only for a specific animal (humans, dogs, sheep, etc.) Releases for children under 12 and pregnant women require special testing, and are made separately. Drugs are released for use only in certain diseases and given dosages, and can only be advertised along these lines. If the FDA has not released a drug for a specific use or disease it does not mean that it isn't of use. It does mean that the FDA has not had reports filed that meet its standards to prove both that the drug is effective for that use, and safe in people with that disease. Although the FDA regulations are both very necessary and reasonable, they do make it very difficult and extremely expensive to get approval to use an old and established drug for a new use, and for new drugs to be marketed.

By tradition and custom, physicians individually often use a drug that has a reasonable safety record in general for a use that isn't FDA approved, but for which the drug is thought to be effective. These decisions are made on an individual basis, patient by patient. Although these practices are generally within the range of what's reasonable by medical tradition, there have been some real abuses of this tradition as well. Current legal opinions have generally held that only the FDA-approved uses are considered "proper" uses of the drug. Although this legal precedent is directly contrary to current medical practice and tradition, it's easy to see why the courts ruled this way. Older drugs (marketed between 1910 and 1956) and drugs already approved have different requirements to remain on the market if problems develop. In the chapters so far, I've tried to give you some idea of which drugs have FDA approval and for what purposes. Since this changes from time to time, you should always check with your own doctor before and during any of these treatments. Remember that FDA lack of approval doesn't mean the treatment is bad, or that the presence of this approval doesn't mean the treatment is certain to be good for you. By and large, I haven't indicated which drugs and treatments are by prescription or not, since you should discuss all of them with your doctor before using them, in all cases.

There are two purposes to the rest of this chapter. The first is to summarize some general features of the treatments for arthritis, since many of them have some things in common. The second is to give you more information on why they work, what they accomplish, what their problems are, and what you should expect to be coming out in the next five years. This information is intended as a supplement to the preceding chapters, not as a replacement for them. It will also give you information you need to evaluate new treatments as they come out, and decide whether they are really what you need.

When talking about treatments for arthritis, the easiest starting place is cures versus hold-the-line treatments.

Arthritis quickly splits into two groups. The curable group has very few kinds of arthritis and currently includes only joint infections and the unusual joint infection, Reiter's disease. The coming development in curable forms of arthritis really is the progressive understanding of the types of infections that can cause arthritis. The real developments, if they are ever made, will be to understand what kinds of infections cause rheumatoid arthritis, fusion arthritis, and the arthritis of intestinal diseases. At this point, it isn't even certain that these types of arthritis are infections at all, though most of the evidence does point in this direction. If they are viral infections, some of the new antibiotics for viruses may prove of use. If they are bacterial, perhaps the long-term use of current antibiotics or ones yet to appear will provide a cure for diseases that, up to now, have not been curable.

The second group, all the other forms of arthritis, have no cure, and are here to stay. The treatment consists of avoiding things that will speed the destruction of the joints and adding chemicals (drugs) that can (1) slow the rate at which the damage progresses, (2) change part of what's going wrong back to normal, and (3) change how we feel pain and discomfort.

Much of what goes wrong in arthritis centers around the chemicals I've called the P-G's. These are a group of chemicals produced on the spot, in the joint or bone at the point of damage. They are made very quickly when damage occurs. For most of them, their effect is also very brief and ceases quickly once the production of these things stops. These chemicals, taken as a group, cause many things to happen, although they aren't the only cause of these things: (1) the pain and swelling of arthritis; (2) the removal and replacement of bone under the teflon caps; (3) starting the destruction of the teflon caps by white blood cells; (4) the activation of white blood cells that destroy bugs infecting a joint; (5) causing damage to the lining of the joints and their blood vessels; (6) and starting the growth of new blood vessels from the joint bag into the bone under the teflon cap.

The extremely wide range of what these chemicals do makes them a prime target for the action of drugs. The fact that most of them disappear soon after they are made means that, if you stop their production, you can also stop their effect. Not all chemicals in the body work that way: some of them, like cortisone, have an effect long after they are gone. The majority of drugs that we use for arthritis work by stopping P-G production. This is not only true of aspirin, Clinoril® and related drugs, but the cortisone-like drugs as well.

Despite the similarities of action, however, not all P-G's are created equally, and not all the medicines against them work in the same places in the body or with the same effectiveness. For example, different P-G's are involved in the activation of the white blood cells, the production of pain, and the removal of bone. The P-G's are made by different chemical factories, too. Each of these factories differs in how sensitive it is to the ability of one drug or another to stop its action. Some drugs are also more effective in some people than others; there do seem to be genetic differences in how well one or another of these drugs stops P-G's of a special type from being made in a person's body.

The P-G's are involved in many other things besides pain and arthritis. They send signals between nerves, control the movement of food through the intestines, regulate blood pressure, and control blood clotting. Our kidney uses them to control the minerals that stay in or leave our body. With all these other things going on, it only stands to reason that some people will have problems with these drugs, again depending largely on a genetic difference in how sensitive each P-G production system is at each part of the body. As a result, aspirin and all its related dozen drugs that stop the production of P-G's work in basically the same way, but have many differences. For some people, the standard drugs won't work well, and others must be tried.

There is a definite order of preference for these aspirin-like drugs that works for most people. Clinoril® is usually at the head of the list. If Clinoril® isn't effective enough, Indocin®, and *phenylbutazone* (or *oxyphenbutazone*), in that order of preference, can be used. However, both of these are more likely to cause ill effects. If Clinoril® has too many undesired effects, next choices in order of preference, are Nalfon® or Tolectin®, Naprosyn®, and Motrin®. Then comes aspirin/buffered aspirin (including Bufferin®, Ascriptin®, and Ecotrin®), *salicylic acid* (Arthropan®, Disalid®, Magan®, and Trilisate®). Note that Empirin®, APC tablets, Anacin®, and Excedrin® are not on the "suitable" list. An exception to this general scheme is Ponstel®. This drug, and one in development (*flufenamic acid*) are unusual in that they not only block the formation of P-G's, but also stop them from acting once they are formed. This double-ended action means that it will act more quickly than the other drugs, and may be more effective for the relief of pain. In general Ponstel® is unusually effective for pain relief, and should be considered for use when the the other drugs are not adequate in this regard. Ponstel® unfortunately has some rare allergic reactions to it, primarily involving the blood count. For this reason, the FDA has not approved it for long-term use. However, the same problems exist with *phenylbutazone* and many of the other drugs used for arthritis. With this caution in mind, Ponstel® may be very useful in certain situations as an addition or alternative to the other aspirin-like drugs. The new derivative, *flufenamic acid*, hasn't shown these problems to date, and may be equal to Clinoril® as a drug for arthritis when it appears in the next decade. One additional word of caution: all the

aspirin-like drugs are slow to act. Aspirin and Ponstel®
are the fastest acting, with *phenylbutazone* next in line.
Even these take one to several days for full effect. Always
try these drugs for more than a few days, and in large
enough amounts, before giving them up. As a last word of
warning, there may be a problem with some types of
buffered aspirin. Recently, there's been some reason to
think that using aluminum-containing antacids (buffers)
regularly causes a progressive loss of calcium from the
bones and weakens the marble in them. At this time, there
isn't enough evidence to say this is so; only that it may be
the case. In view of the seriousness of this for someone
with the wear and tear type of arthritis, people who use
buffered aspirin more than just occasionally should be
sure it doesn't have aluminum in it, until this issue is
settled. Unfortunately, most of the available forms of
buffered aspirin, including Bufferin® and Ascriptin® use
aluminum as the buffer. For occasional use, this seems
OK, but if you use them several times a day, every day,
then use Titralac® or calcium tablets (chewed first) as
your antacid.

Earlier I had mentioned that cortisone and its synthetic
forms like *prednisone* work in the same way as aspirin.
The basis of this is natural chemicals the body can
produce that stop the production of P-G's in any part of
the body, as well as related chemical processes that
aspirin-like drugs can't influence. These chemicals circu-
late freely throughout the body and, once produced, will
stop P-G production in places the cortisone hasn't
reached. The cortisone only serves as a trigger for their
production. Once the cortisone starts their production,
this continues on its own for some hours after the cortisone has disappeared. The cortisone itself actually disap-
pears quickly, although the synthetic forms can stay
around longer. Triggering the production of this material
may not be the only thing cortisone does, but with regard
to arthritis, it is the major action.

Among the materials that stop P-G production, this natural one seems to be the most potent, most far-ranging, and least selective in its effects. Unfortunately, this is the reason cortisone, when used as a drug, has such a wide range of bad effects, and why it isn't possible to make a form of cortisone that is free of the bad effects. The nature of this natural blocker of P-G production isn't known at this time, but learning what this material is and how it works will open the way to a whole new group of drugs for arthritis and other diseases. Any benefits from this discovery are however at least 10 years away.

What are the major problems with cortisone and *prednisone*? For short-term use—a few days to a few weeks — the major problem is in the white blood cells, which are a major defense against infections. They rely on the production of P-G's and related chemicals to trigger and carry out their defensive actions. As a result, people taking *prednisone* tend to get bacterial and fungal infections easily. The more the drug is used, the greater the problem. In particular, reactivation of old TB, staph infections, pneumonia, sinus, and skin infections are the greatest problems.

A second problem is the softening of the bones. Bone is constantly being remodeled and the P-G's are a major chemical signal that the controllers use to regulate this. Although the rate of removal of marble in the bones is decreased by the cortisone, so is the rate of replacement with new marble. The replacement is more severely affected than the removal, and over a period of years, the result is a noticeable loss of marble from the bones. In addition, the cables on which the marble is placed are not made as easily. This combination of things leads to weak bones, easy fractures, and subsequent problems, particularly in the hips and spine.

A third problem, again related to P-G production and shared to some extent with all the aspirin-like drugs, is stomach and intestinal ulcers. The stomach and intestine make a jelly to coat and protect the lining against being eaten by acid and digestive juices from the stomach. The production and release of this material is controlled by P-G's made in the stomach. Cortisone stops this and the lack of the coating can lead to ulcers. In addition, the lack of P-G's probably influences blood supply to the stomach lining, where damage can occur more easily.

A number of other difficulties occur with cortisone use. The skin becomes thin and can tear easily, as can the veins and arteries. Diabetes is usually aggravated by cortisone use, and a mild case can be made quite severe. The use of cortisone and its synthetic forms suppresses the body's own production of these materials, and after a long period of use, the body can't regulate how much cortisone it should produce. As a result, at times of stress when more cortisone is needed, the body runs short of supply. Cataracts can be produced by the prolonged use of cortisone-like drugs. Severe problems with acne, weight gain, and appearance changes can also occur.

How can these problems be lessened? Obviously one way is to use *prednisone* only when necessary. The development of increasingly better drugs for arthritis has made the need for *prednisone* decline a great deal. The drugs to appear in the next five years, *auranofin* and *levamisole*, promise to have an even greater impact in this regard. Unfortunately, *prednisone* may be very necessary for your form of arthritis. *Prednisone* only makes the basic problem in wear and tear arthritis worse and should not be used here. In addition, it is undesirable for Reiter's disease, since this is basically an infection though the severity of joint inflammation may make it necessary. Since we really have to accept the fact that for many people, *prednisone* will be needed, let's go over the ways to lessen most of the undesired effects.

There are two basic things to remember about all the cortisone-like drugs. The first is that all the unwanted effects are related to how much is used, and for how long. The second is that using the drug every second (or third) day greatly reduces the problems with most of these effects. The every other day use is particularly important, and every effort should be made to use the drug in this way. If you take 40 mg of *prednisone* every other day, you'll do yourself less harm than with 15 mg daily, even though the total amount you take per week (140 mg vs. 105 mg) is more. Beyond that, *prednisone* should be used for as short a time as possible, and in as small an amount as possible, even if this means using two or three other drugs as well to keep yourself comfortable.

The shorter the time the cortisone-like drug is in the body, the less serious the bad effects will be. This is the reason that *prednisone* and several similar drugs (*methylprednisone, prednisolone*) are preferred. Their time in the body is short, as it is for natural cortisone. The other drugs (*triamcinalone* or Aristocort®, *betamethasone, dexamethasone* or Decadron®) have progressively longer action in the order listed. For some purposes, these drugs are preferable, but not for arthritis in general. Although shortest in time span, natural cortisone should not be used because it causes severe water and salt retention.

A final factor in avoiding the ill effects of *prednisone*— as strange as this will sound to you—is not to take too little. Normally your body will produce the equivalent (in cortisone) of 7-8 mg of *prednisone* a day. Almost all of this is made between 4 A.M. and noon. For the rest of the day, almost no further cortisone is made. As a treatment for a number of forms of arthritis, some people have used 1-3 mg three times a day, or 5 mg of *prednisone* just in the afternoon. In general, although this may make you feel a bit better, this should not be done. Taking 5-10 mg of *prednisone* a day is not enough to help the arthritis significantly. It also isn't more in total amount than your body makes naturally. But more important, the timing is off. The cortisone is around when it shouldn't be. Your body senses this as an excess of cortisone, and shuts off its own production. As a result, at times of stress, your body frequently won't increase its production of cortisone when it should, which can pose serious problems. In addition, the loss of the no-cortisone period (in the evenings) probably will give you the same undesired effects as listed earlier, though to a milder degree. In general, it's better to use something else, rather than the continuous use of *prednisone* in small amounts.

If aspirin and the related drugs aren't good enough alone, there are several other very useful drugs for many types of arthritis that not only make you feel better, but also help you avoid the use of *prednisone*. When ulcers are a problem, or a true aspirin allergy is present, these drugs are desirable as the first drug to use. As discussed in the chapter on RA, gold injections are available for this purpose. They are useful for RA and the arthritis of psoriasis, but have many undesirable effects. Their moderate degree of effectiveness in relieving the discomfort and slowing the progression of RA gives them some real usefulness. In terms of the way the drugs work, the next one along the line is *penacillamine*. Like the gold injections, this drug works by taking apart the hook and alarm assemblies and by stopping the chemicals released from the white blood cells from working well. *Penacillamine* may have also had some ability to reduce P-G production. It's more effective than the gold drugs in doing these things, and works faster. In addition, its adverse effects go away faster. The range of how much can be used is also quite wide: anywhere from 3 to 12 capsules a day (usual: 3-6). When adverse effects do appear, they can be much worse than with gold, and at least mild undesired effects are common. In approving *penacillamine* for use in arthritis (it's only approved for RA, but is effective in some other forms), the FDA recommends that it should only be used after other measures fail. However, the fact that it shouldn't be used after gold injections for 3-12 months, combined with its fairly fast action suggests that it may be better to use this drug sooner than later, until *aura-nofin* is available.

A group of drugs preferable to either of these are two that work on the white blood cells. As you might recall from Chapter Four, I mentioned a group of drugs for RA that work by stopping the action of the white blood cells. One of these was Cytoxan®. These drugs, you recall, are not a nice choice for any disease. So why would *other* drugs that do the same thing be the preferred ones for RA? Just like the situation with aspirin and cortisone, it's one of degree. Remember that aspirin-like drugs and cortisone basically did the same thing, only cortisone's action was everywhere, and nearly total. The aspirin-like drugs stopped P-G production only in some places and did so only partially. In addition, they didn't affect the substances similar to P-G's (not true P-G's) which cortisone did affect. These "good" white blood cell drugs likewise only do a partial job. Instead of stopping virtually all the actions of the white blood cells, as Cytoxan® does, they partially stop only excessive activities. Plaquanil®, which is currently available, partially prevents the activation of white blood cells to produce lots of hooks, either on their surface or attached to alarms. It also appears able to decrease the release of harmful chemicals from the scavenger white cells that can be caused by activated alarms. It doesn't seem to interfere at all with the "normal" activities of the white blood cells, however. No further work is underway with Plaquanil®-type drugs and no improvements on it are expected in the near future.

Auranofin is much stronger in its effects on the white blood cells than is Plaquanil®, but the idea behind what it does is very much the same. White blood cells usually make copies of themselves when something is near that their hooks (on their surface) will attach to. This is true of either the ones that release hook and alarm assemblies, or the ones that keep the hooks attached to themselves. *Auranofin* largely, though not completely, prevents this. When activated alarms are near a scavenger cell, the scavenger will usually try and eat them and destroy whatever they are attached to. If there are many activated alarms around, the scavenger cell often tosses destructive chemicals out into the surrounding area. This last thing is part of what causes the damage to the body in RA and other forms of arthritis. *Auranofin* almost completely stops this toss-out from happening. By cutting down on the activities of the hook-producing white blood cells, the overall production of hook and alarm assemblies, including rheumatoid factor, is also decreased.

To date, *auranofin* has been very effective for the treatment of RA, with few undesired effects. Unlike the injected gold drugs (whose *only* similarity to *auranofin* is the gold in them) there have been no serious problems to date. *Auranofin* will probably be suitable for use with *penacillamine* if needed, but no tests have been made. The effects of *auranofin* (at the usual dose of 2 mg two or three times a day) start in 3-5 weeks. Benefits would probably appear faster at a higher initial amount, but the risk of undesired effects is also greater. *Auranofin* remains in the body for several months after it is stopped, and its benefits likewise continue to some extent for that time. *Auranofin,* when released, will be one of the best available treatments for RA and other forms of arthritis. At this time, several serious questions remain about it. First, the effect of *auranofin* on suppressor cells, which are probably underactive in RA, is unknown. It probably decreases their action, which is an undesirable effect. Second, *auranofin* causes some depression of our defenses against infection. With Plaquanil®, a similar action has not proved to be a problem. Whether it will be with *auranofin* or not isn't certain yet. *Auranofin* appears selective enough in what it does to avoid this problem, still, the proof is lacking. Third, the most potent drugs that affect the white blood cells, like Cytoxan®, have posed a problem with the late development of cancer, because of these effects. Again, this doesn't seem to be a problem with *auranofin*, but at this time, we just don't know its effects on the white blood cells that help prevent cancer. These cells are, incidentally, different from those discussed so far in this book. Fourth, all trials to date have used *auranofin* for less than a year's time. The long-term safety of the drug isn't known yet, even though no problems are expected at this time.

If *auranofin* proves suitable for use, it will be a desirable drug for far more than just RA. Again unlike the gold injections, but like Plaquanil®, *auranofin* has shown itself to be effective for inflammation in general, as well as for some types of allergic reactions. It will probably prove to be useful for most of the diseases discussed in this book, including gout and the other inflammatory types of arthritis (but not wear arthritis) as well as the look-alikes for RA (Chapter Five). In addition, it will probably be useful for asthma, and some skin diseases. It could be tried in the arthritis of *psoriasis* as well. Lately there has been some indication that it may be of limited use in the treatment of some types of cancer.

One of the possibilities for both *penacillamine* and *auranofin* is in a form of arthritis that hasn't been really discussed in this book: joint infections. When bacteria infect a joint, they and the white blood cells that fight them release chemicals into the joint fluid that eat into and try to destroy the joint. As a result, serious and permanent joint damage often occurs, even with prompt treatment. Since *penacillamine* can inactivate some of these chemicals, and *auranofin* can prevent their release from the white blood cells, both of these drugs may be quite valuable when used in conjunction with antibiotics for joint infections. This is especially so in Reiter's disease (Chapter Five).

The drugs that ultimately suppress the white blood cells were discussed in the chapter on RA. These drugs, Cytoxan®, Imuran®, and (for *psoriasis*) *methotrexate* can cause near total suppression of white blood cell action. As mentioned, these drugs are extremely effective for most inflammatory diseases, over the short run. They are also the most undesirable of all the drugs used and are generally only used along with *prednisone*. At this time, their use is limited to rapidly progressive RA, severe non-arthritis problems that go along with RA, the severe arthritis that can occur in *psoriasis*, and serious look-alikes for RA. A few new drugs are under development as replacements to these, but the improvements that are expected aren't great. Basically, drugs of this general type offer an alternative to severe, uncontrollable illness, and to prolonged use of large amounts of *prednisone*. Regrettably, sometimes RA and other diseases are severe enough to require their use. When they really are needed, it's best to use them sooner than later, since *they can only prevent damage, not repair it.* Hopefully, developments like *auranofin* and *levamisole* will make their use increasingly unnecessary.

On the other side of the coin are the drugs that stimulate the white blood cells. These drugs show a tremendous potential for RA and other forms of arthritis (except wear and tear) for two reasons. The first is they are able to help halt the joint disease and destruction without stopping the body's normal defenses. The second is that RA and related forms of arthritis are due sometimes to chronic infections. These drugs, while helping the arthritis, also help the body rid itself of the infection. Many of the other drugs available do exactly the opposite for any possible underlying infection.

One of these drugs, Tagamet®, is readily available, but not specifically approved for use in RA and related diseases. Like the other drugs, it stimulates more types of white blood cells than just the suppressor cells. As a result, at times it may make inflammation worse rather than better, depending on what's causing it. In addition, it won't always stimulate the white blood cells, but works primarily when their action is being stopped or held back by something else. The drug is extremely free of ill effects, and quick-acting. If it does make the situation worse (which doesn't happen often), you'll know quickly and can expect things to return to the way they were soon after you stop taking it. Experience with Tagamet® in arthritis is very limited, and it's hard to say just how useful it will prove to be. It does appear to be at least moderately effective, though, and is the only drug in this group marketed for human use at this time.

The second drug of this type, *levamisole* (Ripercol®), is only approved for use in some animals at this time but will probably be available for human use in the early 1980s. Although this drug works on the white blood cells in a different way from Tagamet®, it also stimulates the suppressor cells as well as other white blood cells in the body. Like Tagamet®, most of its effects are felt only when the white blood cells are being kept less active by something else. Most of the time, *levamisole* won't raise the activity of the white blood cells above normal. The drug has been tried in RA, fusion arthritis, and the look-alikes for RA (like *lupus*). In each disease, it has been helpful for 60-80% of the people who used it. In general, the improvement has been equal to that achieved with *auranofin*, but occurs faster. The main problem with it have been skin rash and low blood count. A few children with RA and juvenile RA have had serious additional problems, as noted in Chapter Four. Unlike Tagamet®, whose effect comes and goes quickly, *levamisole's* effect lasts for some time after the drug is stopped. As a result, the most useful way of taking the drug has been once every 3-7 days. This way of taking it also seems to remove the blood count problem fairly well. Levamisole seems to have no effect on the white blood cells usually involved in preventing cancer.

A last drug along these lines, still in early experimental stages, is tilorone. This drug, unlike Tagamet® and levamisole, seems to stimulate the white blood cells that make hook and alarm assemblies as well as the ones that have only surface hooks. Since it isn't certain that it can stimulate suppressor cells, the usefulness of tilorone isn't clear. Unlike the first two, this drug may also be able to stimulate the white blood cells to a more than normal level of activity.

At this time, the development of this general group of drugs is probably the most significant advance in the treatment of RA, and many other inflammatory diseases. Over the coming decade, drugs like auranofin and levamisole (although not necessarily those particular ones) will probably be the first choice for treatment of these diseases. Even if a complete cure is discovered for RA and other diseases, these drugs will still be useful to prevent damage to the body while the cure is going on.

None of the drugs mentioned so far are just pain relievers. All of them, in addition to relieving pain, work primarily on stopping the process that causes the pain. Not all medicines that relieve pain work that way. Tylenol® lessens the feeling of pain without affecting anything that causes it. Morphine and codeine do this, too. At this time, we don't really know how Tylenol® works, though we do know some of the basics of how morphine and codeine operate. It has to do with how we feel pain.

When we feel something, that "feeling" starts out as an electrical signal from the point that's being touched, stung, hit or whatever. That bit of electricity travels along our body's version of an electric wire, and after going through a number of switches, reaches our brain. We don't sense the arrival of the signal yet, though. When the signal first reaches our brain, it is "processed" before we even know it's there. Depending on whether we're awake or asleep, happy or sad, doing something or not, that signal either is strengthened or weakened. It may be turned off entirely or become extremely strong. Depending on what other signals have already arrived, it may have a painful feel added on or not. While all this is going on, that signal also triggers off other messages to the muscles and other parts of the body. Based on that original signal before we feel anything, our brain triggers our body to do something. This is called a reflex. Finally, after all this is done, that signal—modified and refined—is sent higher up in the brain, and we feel it. Our feeling is like a phone conversation, over true electrical wires, between the place where the feeling starts and the brain. It's not a direct connection. At several places in between, the conversation is tapped into it. This triggers things to happen even before we realize it's taking place. And the conversation is changed to some extent, before we realize what's going on. This last process, which takes place on the "lower levels" of the brain, is the basis of how narcotics relieve pain without reducing inflammation. These drugs put in extra signals that relieve the pain we feel. Some people would say that these drugs don't get rid of pain, they just mask it. According to our understanding of what pain is to begin with, that's just playing with words. Pain can be removed in three different ways: The cause can be eliminated, the signal lines can be shut down, or the interpretation of the feeling as pain can go. Most of the drugs mentioned so far do the first thing; anesthetics, like Novocaine® and ether, do the second; the narcotics do the last.

Our body naturally regulates the amount of pain we

feel, by producing natural narcotics within our brain. These chemicals are made in a different way than morphine, but they work in exactly the same way. Depending on how much is present, and where in the brain they are at any time, what we sense as painful or not changes. These natural narcotics, called *endorphins,* have been suspected as present for a long time, but were discovered only a few years ago. Now that we know where these materials are, what they are made of, and where they work, it will be possible to make new, narcotic drugs that give better pain relief, with less sleepiness, nausea, constipation, confusion, and above all, less addiction than narcotics now available. The only unfortunate thing is that the introduction of these drugs to the market is ten years away.

With most of the forms of arthritis discussed in this book, there's a problem with lubrication of the joint. With RA and related diseases, a defective lubricant is produced. With wear arthritis, there is a thinning of the teflon cap which doesn't lubricate itself properly as a result. In joints damaged by old injury or infection, again destruction of part of the teflon cap prevents good lubrication and leads to rapid wear. Obviously, one thing that would be useful is a joint lubricant that could be injected into the joint and left there. At the present time, nothing like that is available. However, another approach has been to use plates of real Teflon® as caps on the bones, and to just replace them periodically. This saves a complete replacement of the joint, and often works well. Teflon® isn't perfect though, because it is a glass: a liquid that thinks it's a solid. With repeated pressure it becomes brittle and can form small breaks and chips. Other plastics have been more promising as self-lubricating artificial joint surfaces, but this work is still experimental. All the plastics used so far have a problem of long-term durability. As new plastics and metal alloys are developed though, the replacement of the "teflon" caps on the bones remains a real possibility for the future. In general, it's much more desirable for many reasons to just replace the teflon cap at the ends of the bones that form the joint, than to replace the entire joint, bone and all. This last is done in the usual joint replacement.

For wear arthritis, one drug has appeared that shows some potential for arresting some aspects of the disease. The basic process in wear arthritis, you recall, is repeated fracture and removal of bone under the joint, without proper replacement of the bone afterwards. In addition, extra bone is put in place in areas where it shouldn't be, forming the spurs of this type of arthritis. A new drug, Didronel®, is able to decrease the removal of bone and prevent it from being added to new areas that are forming spurs. The drug is currently used for this general purpose in a different problem: Paget's disease, also mentioned in the second chapter. The amount of Didronel® that might be useful in wear arthritis is much lower than that used in Paget's disease. Experience with Didronel® in wear arthritis is very limited, and the correct dosage in this disease isn't clear yet, so it can't be used "blindly." Too much of it will lead to weakening of the bones, and only worsen the wear arthritis, so real care must be taken. However, the potential is obviously there for this drug to slow or halt the progression of at least spur formation in this type of arthritis, if it is used at the right dosage. As mentioned in Chapter Two, some tests are currently available to help in this respect. Of course, Didronel® has not received FDA approval for use in arthritis.

All the treatments so far in this chapter are designed to preserve function in the joints, and keep them from becoming further damaged. However, in some people, the joints do become so badly damaged that they just can't be used at all. Sometimes the joint surfaces (teflon faces) become so worn that the bone underneath them just rubs directly against the bone on the other side of the joint. The pain becomes so great that the joint just can't be used. When this happens, often the joint fuses on its own, and a solid weld forms across what used to be a joint. Sometimes the cables that hold the joint together (ligaments) become quite weak and loose as well. The joint then becomes a floppy link that can't support any weight, and just wiggles about. In this situation, unfortunately, the bones don't fuse, but just hang loosely. In these circumstances there really is no joint left to preserve and the only alternative is joint replacement, if possible. Some artificial joints are available at this time, and more are being developed for future use. What do these joint replacements consist of, and where can they be used? When should they be used?

Before going into the uses of these joint replacements, let me begin by saying that they aren't for everybody, or every joint affected by arthritis. Since all of these replacements are not "self-renewing" the way our natural joints are, they have a limited lifespan on their own: sometimes ten years, sometimes much less. There are also problems with them, and these differ depending on which joint replacement one is talking about. Joint replacements are generally a last resort, used for a joint that is pretty much totally destroyed. They're for use by a person who would profit from a replacement with a limited "lifespan."

The most successful joint replacement by far has been the hip joint. This success has been quite recent. People have attempted hip replacements since the late 1880s. Real success began only in the late 1950s and early 1960s, and was due to developments in special plastics that were essentially self-lubricating. At this time, hip replacements give people who have lost nearly all use of the hip or who have extreme pain in the hip the ability to walk and move about freely. The recovery period after a hip joint replacement is usually short. The replacement lasts about ten years and includes the upper part of the leg bone and part of the pelvic bone as well. When needed, a second or third replacement is usually successful as well. In older people following a hip fracture, a joint replacement is usually done since the chances of surviving and walking again are better than after a pinning of the fracture. The hip replacements are usually not of use in people who have frequent dislocations of the hip, since this still can occur easily after the replacement. Hip replacement is particularly of use in people who lose the use of the hip from wear arthritis, fusion arthritis (even though young), and premature wear arthritis from congenital hip problems and juvenile RA. It is of some, though much less use for people with severe RA. Usually the knee, ankle, and foot are also badly affected in this situation, and hip replacement then can contribute little overall.

There are a number of problems with blood clot formation following the operation, and a low but significant rate of death during the operation itself. The operation is generally not done in the presence of infection (which also occurs after 1-2% of the hip operations) with present methods. The use of antibiotics incorporated in the cement that holds the joint in place, however, may make this type of joint replacement possible even in the event of infection, if it is partially controlled first.

The knee is the next common joint replacement. There are a number of models of replacements used, generally depending on how much of the bone has been destroyed and how weak the ligaments are. Unlike the hip, the ends of the bones that form the joint normally aren't removed. To get any of these replacement joints to work, a person must be at a reasonable weight before the replacement, or the knees just won't take the strain. Unlike the situation with the hip, knee joint replacement is primarily of use when the joint is frozen. It isn't of use as a treatment for pain or weak ligaments. The recovery from surgery is longer and more difficult. Normal use of the knee is never restored; at best, one gets about 30% of normal use. Like the hip joint, this replacement is not done in the presence of infection. Being a rolling block joint, the success of this replacement depends on the strength of the muscles and cables around the knee that hold it together. If these are weak, the replacement works poorly until they are strengthened. As with the hip, blood clots and infections are a problem in 2-5% of these replacements. When the cable support for the knee is extremely weak and the knee buckles easily, a hinge joint can be used for replacement. This type of joint wears out quickly, however, and it is used little.*

The other replacement joints don't try to duplicate the way our joints work naturally, as the knee and hip replacements do. Instead, they are a piece of very flexible silicone rubber, which our body tolerates well. These joints are basically a rubber pad, with ends that go into the bone above and below the joint. This forms a flexible hinge for the bones involved. These joints can be used in the feet, hands, fingers, some of the bones of the wrist, and the elbow. In each case the replacement works in the same way.

The life of the artificial joint is limited by the rubber's ability to withstand constant bending, and runs from 5 to 10 years. The rubber isn't stiff enough to stabilize a weak

------

*The real story on blood clots forming during joint replacements is actually quite complicated. The percentages given in the text refer to serious or life-threatening blood clots only. These are the figures quoted by most physicians. Actually, if the clots are looked for carefully, 50-90% of the people with hip and knee replacements develop clots, UNLESS effective drug treatments are used to prevent their formation. The actual percentage depends on the details of the replacement and the condition of the patient who is having it done. Obviously, only 10-20% of the clots that do form are actually considered serious by the physicians doing the replacements.

and floppy joint. If this is the problem, usually the bones across the joint are fused by surgery. The rubber joints are useful only if the cables and muscles around the joint can hold it steady. Changes in the design of these joints are constantly being made, and better forms of silicone rubber are being developed. As with the other replacement joints, problems with infection occur, but blood clots don't form too often afterwards.

Two completely new types of plastics have been developed by Union Carbide and DuPont that have many properties that make them very promising for use in artificial joints. This is a development that won't appear for our use for some time.

Most often, joint replacement is something primarily for older adults, but there are several exceptions to this. Younger people with severe hip problems from fusion arthritis, RA, or congenital hip malformation probably should have hip replacements done sooner than later. A repeat replacement can be done in ten years or so, as needed. Also, finger joint replacements are suitable for younger people with RA, *psoriasis,* and other forms of severe hand arthritis.

In general, though, you must remember that the joint replacements are not a cure for arthritis, but only an alternative to loss of use from total joint destruction. Usually they should not be done in growing children, since once the joint is replaced, the bone won't grow further. Also, replacing a joint can't change the basic disease causing the arthritis.

Some Common Questions

One of the big questions people with arthritis have is: What exercises can I do to cure the arthritis? There aren't any that will cure it. Exercises really can do only two things to benefit your arthritis. The first is they keep the joint from freezing, fixed in one position. They do this two ways. (1) They keep stretching and relaxing the muscles and tendons. Normally this happens all the time as we move about, both while awake and asleep. However when arthritis involves a joint, people tend not to move the bones that make up the joint. This causes the muscles and tendons to shorten, locking the joint in place. (2) In addition, the damage in the joint tends to form a cement from the lubricating fluid that glues the joint fixed in one position. By moving the joint frequently, the cement is constantly being broken, and the joint can't freeze as easily.

The other thing that exercise does is keep the joint lubricated. Remember that how much lubricant is made depends on the activity of the joint. If the joint isn't used at all, little lubricant is made. So some amount of activity and exercise is needed just to preserve this basic lubrication. This usually happens with normal activity, but some people with arthritis are so inactive that there isn't enough movement at the joints to preserve the lubrication.

Exercise is needed for one other reason, not directly related to helping the arthritis itself. The amount of marble in the bone is controlled by how much stress the bone endures, and how much weight is pressing on it. When an arm or leg isn't used much, the electrical forces in the bones aren't produced, and the bone can lose marble rapidly. Since P-G's are involved and can cause pain, this loss of marble can be painful enough to further prevent the arm or leg from being used. This, in turn, leads to still more loss of bone mineral and more pain. In the end, this can create the "reflex sympathetic dystrophy" discussed earlier in Chapter 2.

The exercises for arthritis are all intended to do several things. First, the joints should be moved through as wide a range as possible, to keep the muscles and tendons from shortening and break any glued spots within the joint.

Second, a small or moderate amount of weight or force should be involved but not very heavy lifting. This way, the bone is at least partially prevented from losing its marble, and some lubricant is stimulated, but no excessive stress is placed on the joint to cause extra wear. Third, frequent exercises for a short period are better than one long, rare session. Finally, any exercise that puts the joint under sudden pressure or stress should be avoided. The exercises themselves are discussed in Chapter 2, but they apply to all types of arthritis. Remember: They won't cure anything, they won't stop the arthritis from progressing, and they won't help the pain. No exercises can do that. Only the medicines discussed earlier can.

Another treatment that some people have turned to for arthritis is vitamins. It's true that a lack of certain vitamins can cause bone disease (not arthritis), but no vitamin is of use in treating arthritis. The same applies for all diets: there just isn't any diet that will really help for arthritis. The only relationship between the two is that in an occasional instance, a high-iron diet can cause a special type of arthritis. The problem, called *hemochromatosis*, is discussed earlier in the book. The reason for this lack of help from diet is clear if you think about what we really get from vitamins and diet. Our diets have nothing magic about them. We eat food for several reasons. A source of energy to move and heat our bodies, and enable our brains to work; a source of vitamins, which I'll go into in a minute; and a source of building blocks to make bones, skin, and internal parts. As you've seen in the preceding chapters, *no type of arthritis is the result of a lack of building blocks or energy.* The problems are really entirely different from that, and won't be helped by providing more of these things. There are enough already. If you need 10,000 bricks to make a house, having 30,000 on the lot won't help build it any faster than 11,000. Having three electrical outlets side-by-side for one lamp won't help you any more so than one or two outlets would.

So more energy and building blocks won't help. What about the vitamins? This all centers on what the vitamins really do. They are not medicines or drugs. *Vitamins won't cure any illnesses in most of us, or prevent diseases in the usual sense.* Sure, there are illnesses that are the result of a complete lack of vitamins. But that's like saying a light bulb is sick because the fuse is missing. Like the fuse, the vitamin really should have been there to begin with. The disease that results from a lack of vitamins is really something that shouldn't happen in the first place.

Vitamins, except for one, are all a type of chemical called a catalyst. Catalysts are chemicals that "let things happen" at a much faster rate or pace than they normally could. The "catalytic converter" on a car is an example of a catalyst. These converters take oxygen and carbon monoxide (a poisonous gas), and combine them to make carbon dioxide, a harmless gas. The converter is coated on the inside with beads of a special metal that help the oxygen and carbon dioxide combine at a fast pace. Normally, they barely combine at all. Ideally, the catalyst (the special metal in the converter) isn't used up in the process. Putting a dozen converters in the back seat of the car won't make the exhaust any cleaner, but it will be expensive. Vitamins are the same. They aren't burned up, or used up in their job. A tiny amount, less than a speck of dust, is lost each day by washout, and that's all that needs to be replaced every day in adults. Children need to take more vitamins in order to build up a stockpile. For all the claims that are made, taking more vitamins won't heal infections, cure colds, take care of arthritis, increase strength, or do anything other than what goes on normally.

Of course, there are a few exceptions. For extremely

rare diseases, specific vitamins have been useful as drugs. But these occasions are very uncommon. When they do occur, one special vitamin in very large amounts is needed, not many vitamins in moderate amounts. But remember, these diseases are very rare and very special. The big exception to all this is vitamin D, which is not a catalyst at all. It's the start of a material that the body makes for use as a chemical signal or message. The body starts with vitamin D, and makes it into two other chemicals that act as messengers. One of them tells the intestine how much calcium to take into the body. The other tells the bone how much marble to lay down. Vitamin D with calcium has been used as a treatment for a disease where the bones weaken due to lack of marble (osteoporosis). However, this disease is not a form of arthritis, and vitamin D and calcium are not as good as treatments for any form of arthritis. Besides, large amounts of vitamin D can be deadly.

What about arthritis treatments you can buy "over the counter" at a drug store or supermarket? Only two of these are good for arthritis: aspirin (plain or buffered) and *salicyclic acid* (Arthropan®). These drugs are discussed fully in this book. *Do not make regular use of any drug that contains phenacetin or acetaminophen for your arthritis.* Drugs containing these should only be used occasionally. The linaments, rub-on lotions, and ointments all use a drug similar to aspirin and *salicylic acid* (methyl salicylate or oil of wintergreen). Some also have menthol, which doesn't do anything. What you're doing with these is rubbing aspirin on the skin, and letting it soak into the ligaments and tendons. The only problem is that the drug isn't aspirin and is very irritating to the skin. It also won't work as well as the oral medicines. So, the ointments and rub-ons aren't recommended. They are OK for occasional use, if you like them, but don't use them often. Frequent irritation and damage to the skin of that sort can cause real problems. Also don't try to drink them. That's often fatal.

Many people each year turn to black market drugs and foreign "magic cure" clinics for arthritis. Most of these drugs are either *prednisone* (or another form of cortisone) or *phenylbutazone*, which have been discussed already, and are not recommended. They are particularly dangerous in the large amounts that are used at these clinics and in the black market pills.

Are there drugs coming out that are really strong pain-relievers but not narcotic? There aren't any nonprescription drugs of that sort in the works at this time. The nonnarcotic drugs that are significantly stronger than Tylenol® for pain relief are all out of the aspirinlike drug family. Although all of these drugs, including aspirin itself, are good at relieving pain, some seem more effective than the others.

One is Ponstel®, discussed earlier, and another is a related drug, Meclomen®, which was released in mid-1980. Another one is Zomax®, which is expected to be released soon. Zomax®, is chemically related to Tolectin®, but its undesirable effects are more similar to those of Clinoril®. However, its pain-relieving effectiveness appears comparable to morphine injections in some situations. Thus, Zomax® appears to be substantially better than other aspirinlike drugs as a pain-reliever. Although it appears safe for short-term use (days to weeks), its safety for long-term, day-after-day use hasn't been established yet. As a result, its role in the treatment of arthritis isn't clear. At least it will be of significant help for the pain from brief flare-ups of arthritis. Since Zomax® isn't a narcotic, it isn't likely to be habit forming, and tests for that problem haven't shown any liability for addiction.

A number of magic cure clinics advertise a new wonder drug for arthritis called DMSO (dimethylsulfoxide). This drug has been around for many years, and its good and bad sides are well known. DMSO and a drug mentioned earlier, colchicine, work basically the same way. However, their effects on the body differ somewhat, because the drugs can't go to the same places, and they hang around for different amounts of time once they do get where they are going.

The actions of both drugs center around a type of conveyor-belt system that the body has in virtually all of its cells. The operation of the belt system is important for all cells and essential for the survival of many of them in the long run. However, most cells can stand a brief interruption of the belt system quite well. These belts are something like the tread or tracks on a bulldozer: Many links are put together, and each has a blade or plate of steel that can bite into the dirt for traction. The belts in our cells are a bit different in one important way. On the bulldozer, the belt moves. In our cells, the belt stands still (usually). Instead, the blades push things along the course of the belt. In regard to arthritis, the white blood cells use these belts when they pick up bugs and particles and destroy them. So the belts are essential in producing inflammation when white blood cells are involved. The ability to stop these belts from working makes colchicine and DMSO effective antiinflammatory agents. Both of them cause the links of the belts to fall apart, as long as the drug is present. When the drug is gone, the links go back together on their own, and things start up again.

Colchicine is limited in effectiveness because it is very sticky. If taken as a pill, most of it stays in the stomach and intestines, which it can injure easily. If it enters a vein, most of it remains in the vein and ends up in the liver, which also can be injured by the drug. Fortunately, it cannot reach the brain to affect the nerves there. As a result of this ability to damage the body, very little colchicine can be given, and this limits its effectiveness as a drug. DMSO, on the other hand, enters the body immediately wherever it's given (skin, lungs, stomach, by vein) and easily goes everywhere, including the brain. There is no way to confine it to one spot. Anywhere it goes, it prevents the white blood cells from carrying out an inflammatory reaction by stopping their conveyor belt system. Unlike colchicine, it isn't sticky and leaves (via the lungs and skin) reasonably quickly. Because it is distributed so well, relatively large amounts can be used as a drug without serious effects from a one-time use. However, its free penetration to the brain and nerves is perhaps the most serious problem with repeated use. The nerves, including the brain itself, rely on the belt system to carry supplies down the very long lengths of tubing that make up their "phone lines." If this system is stopped for a brief time, no harm results. But if the interruption is prolonged or repeated, the nerves are badly damaged and can die. In addition, serious liver and lung damage results. This type of problem with the nerves and liver has appeared with long-term use of colchicine, but not in the brain (since colchicine can't get there). In addition, cataracts have been a problem in the eyes of some animals with repeated use of DMSO. Either single-time or repeated use can also cause water loss from the body (a diuretic effect).

With these problems in mind, it's probably wise that the FDA has approved DMSO for human use only in certain diseases where it will be used only once. Obviously, general use for arthritis, where repeated doses over long periods of time are needed, isn't a good idea. Quite literally, you'd lose your mind if you did. However, there are a few diseases where repeated use may be justified, when no other treatment is effective at all or where current treatments are more dangerous than DMSO. Obviously, considering how it works, DMSO can never be a cure either for arthritis or for other diseases for which it has been suggested, unless the basic cause of the problem is a one-time accident or injury. DMSO is FDA approved for arthritic conditions in some animals at this time. But remember, most animals don't live nearly as long as we do, and there is much less concern about the long-term brain power of a race horse than there is for a person.

If you do go to a clinic that recommends DMSO, remember that a number of places have been advertising DMSO but give a form of cortisone or phenylbutazone instead. DMSO comes only as a clear liquid, never as a pill. Also, within two minutes of taking it, your breath will smell like garlic or bitter almonds. If this doesn't happen, you haven't taken DMSO. Although repeated use of DMSO is not recommended for arthritis, routine use of large amounts of drugs similar to cortisone or phenylbutazone is usually not advisable either. If the DMSO is applied to the skin over a joint, the skin must be cleaned thoroughly first (including removal of any soap) since DMSO will carry anything on the skin directly into the blood and joint itself.

Does this mean DMSO isn't of any use for arthritis? Not really. A number of problems can come up in arthritis where a once-only or occasional use of the drug can be helpful. These would include sprains, knee (Baker's) cysts, and sudden joint swelling from any arthritic problem that is severe but infrequent. In large part DMSO could serve in the role once advocated for cortisone injections into joints and tendons, with less damage than these did in the past. For these uses it could be applied on the skin rather than injected. The reactions from DMSO in such instances would be mild ones: pain and stinging upon first application and the possible occurence of hives. The currently available drug preparation of DMSO (50% DMSO in water) may prove suitable for these uses. In addition to these conditions there are rare, arthritis-associated problems and common diseases having nothing to do with arthritis for which there is either no other treatment than

DMSO or only more dangerous ones. It is for those problems that DMSO may be used eventually.

Again, remember that the FDA has recommended that DMSO should only be used for one, uncommon bladder problem. The uses discussed above are only possible places where DMSO may prove to be helpful and are not recommended for treating these problems.

When new treatments for arthritis appear on the market, they're worth your time to check into. There are an incredible number of frauds and fakes in the world, particularly with arthritis, so be careful, and try to think things through before you try them. Some of the wonder treatments that have hit the market in the past few years have been particularly dangerous, and more are certain to follow.

Index

This index uses common names for medical terms and trade names for specific drugs as a point of reference. The medical term for the common name follows in parenthesis as does the generic name of a drug. If you look up a medical term in the index, you will be referred to the entry under its common name.

When using this index to obtain information about diseases and their treatments, remember that statements regarding the causes of a disease and the suggested treatments are matters of medical opinion; they are not fact. The opinions are presented as general statements, intended as items of general information, and may or may not apply to any specific person or his illness.